Effective Language
in Health and Social Work

Effective Language in Health and Social Work

Richard Pugh

North East Wales Institute,
Wrexham, Wales, UK

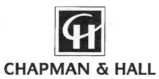

CHAPMAN & HALL

London · Glasgow · Weinheim · New York · Tokyo · Melbourne · Madras

Published by Chapman & Hall, 2–6 Boundary Row, London SE1 8HN, UK

Chapman & Hall, 2–6 Boundary Row, London SE1 8HN, UK

Blackie Academic & Professional, Wester Cleddens Road, Bishopbriggs, Glasgow G64 2NZ, UK

Chapman & Hall GmbH, Pappelallee 3, 69469 Weinheim, Germany

Chapman & Hall USA, 115 Fifth Avenue, New York, NY 10003, USA

Chapman & Hall Japan, ITP-Japan, Kyowa Building, 3F, 2-2-1 Hirakawacho, Chiyoda-ku, Tokyo 102, Japan

Chapman & Hall Australia, 102 Dodds Street, South Melbourne, Victoria 3205, Australia

Chapman & Hall India, R. Seshadri, 32 Second Main Road, CIT East, Madras 600 035, India

Distributed in the USA and Canada by Singular Publishing Group Inc., 4284 41st Street, San Diego, California 92105

First edition 1996

© 1996 Richard Pugh

Typeset in Times 10/12pt by Saxon Graphics Ltd

Printed in Great Britain by Page Bros, (Norwich) Ltd

ISBN 0 412 56730 X   1 56593 324 9 (USA)

A catalogue record for this book is available from the British Library

Library of Congress Catalog Card Number: 95-71376

♾ Printed on permanent acid-free text paper, manufactured in accordance with ANSI/NISO Z39.48-1992 and ANSI/NISO Z39.48-1984 (Permanence of Paper).

Contents

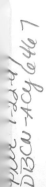

Preface

The stimulus for this book began when I, a monoglot English speaker, was involved in bilingual interviews for candidates for a social work course in North Wales. During the interviews, in which the first half was conducted in Welsh and the second half in English, it was apparent how much more comfortable and at ease the prospective students were when speaking Welsh. They relaxed physically, their conversation became more confident and they were altogether less anxious. I began to wonder what was going on, when apparently capable students who had been educated in English or bilingually, showed such marked difference according to the language they were using. From this developed not simply an interest in the Welsh language, but a broader curiosity about what part language played in social relations and especially in the construction of personal identity within minority groups.

As I read and researched the subject, the idea for this book was further developed by two other discoveries. The first, was that although many academic fields studied language, the most relevant texts from linguistics and sociolinguistics were often fairly inaccessible. Frequently, the books and articles that I sought were highly specialized with limited circulation, and having found them, were initially quite daunting for the casual reader. An additional difficulty was that the professional language of linguistics, which like all academic study struggles to capture and describe ideas with precision, has developed a vocabulary of abbreviations, acronyms and technical terms which arguably results in one of the most esoteric and stylized of discourses within the social sciences. The second discovery was that there seemed to be little direct application of the potentially valuable insights of linguistics within the professional literature for students and practitioners within the human services, such as nursing, social work and teaching.

I hope this book makes a useful contribution to the dissemination, popularization and application of this knowledge. Whilst I have sought to clarify the sometimes complex ideas and intricate distinctions, I hope that this has not led to oversimplification nor is misinterpreted as thus, though inevitably some subtleties are always lost. Furthermore, the selective application of ideas by virtue of their relevance to practice, should not lead the reader to suppose that I have intended to misrepresent the range of debate within linguistics. This book is an introductory text which is intended to stimulate the reader to consider the propositions advanced, and to encourage further exploration and development of the practical application of the subject.

Acknowledgements

Steven Box once noted that, while it was customary to acknowledge the unstinting advice and support of friends, colleagues, publishers and one's long-suffering spouse without whom the manuscript would never have emerged, he felt unable to do so since he was without the necessary stage props, and had thus produced the book virtually single-handed. While it is true that no novice author such as myself ever really appreciates, before they accept the publisher's contract, just how many hours and days they will spend in solitary toil, I have been fortunate in having had good advice and support from start to finish. Whether I have fully accepted or even understood it is of course another matter.

Thus, I have a few dues to pay. To Jo Campling for her sound advice and robust common sense in getting the thing going in the first place. To my colleague Neil Thompson for his careful advice and the loan of many source texts. To Sian Wyn Siencyn, Susan Thompson and Hywel Williams for reading and commenting on the draft manuscript. Lastly to Bridgett Pugh, who put up with living in a cowshed and caravan while we attempted to build a house, and patiently (or fairly so!) waited for me to finish writing so that the usual comforts of home life, such as electricity and an indoor toilet, could be acquired.

Finally, thanks are due to Geoff Beattie, Andrew Ellis, and David Crystal for permission to reproduce amended versions of their diagrams.

Introduction

The purpose of this book is to review and consider some of the vast range of formal knowledge about language and language variation, and to identify its relevance for workers in the health and welfare services. Much of this formal knowledge is not easily accessible for people who are not directly involved in the study of language; it is my aim in this book to broaden the circulation of this work and to begin to synthesize the most useful elements into the development of an antidiscriminatory approach to education and practice. As this is intended as an introductory text, a thorough review of complex ideas and theories, such as dualism, discourse analysis, structuration, and so on, is beyond its scope. In order to make many of the core ideas accessible, I have inevitably had to simplify complex theories, some of which raise fundamental questions about the philosophy, social psychology and the sociology of knowledge, but I have tried not to oversimplify nor lose sight of the spirit of the original work. I would recommend readers whose interest is stimulated by these ideas to explore the literature themselves; this is one of the most fascinating and fast-developing areas of academic research and there is much for us to absorb and apply.

This is not the first book within the human service field that recognizes the significance of language: classic texts such as *The Client Speaks* (Mayer and Timms, 1970), and the extensive literature on counselling and casework, have already done this. It is, however, probably the first text that attempts to integrate such a broad range of material drawn from anthropology, linguistics, sociolinguistics, nursing, philosophy, psychology, social work and sociology for the practical purpose of improving health and welfare practice. Whether it succeeds in this ambitious aim is for the reader to decide. Nevertheless, I hope that every reader will find something of interest in this book and if it stimulates the debate on practice, if only to contest my propositions, then it will have partly achieved its purpose.

Language is one of those concepts that most people believe they instinctively understand but which upon reflection prove surprisingly difficult to define accurately. This book is mainly concerned with the spoken language used in everyday conversation, but follows the normal practice of using the word 'language' to refer to a particular language and as a generic word for all languages; it also refers to both written and signed forms. Linguistics conventionally refers to the study or science of language; though it may appear to be a rather narrow discipline, having considerable overlap with other fields such as psychology and philosophy, there is a surprising range of diversity within it. Some writers have attempted to identify the structures that underpin the human capacity for language (Chomsky, 1968); others have attempted to identify the universal characteristics of languages (Hockett, 1958), while others have sought to study languages as abstract systems of signs that symbolize meaning (Katz, 1981). The term 'sociolinguistics' is usually reserved for the study of the relationship between language and society. Typically the focus is on language as it is used rather than language as a self-contained system. Sociolinguistics is thus concerned with linguistic variation between people and groups, variations that may indicate differences in perception, meaning, identity, status and power. In practice, the distinction between linguistics and sociolinguistics is not rigidly observed, but since this book is primarily concerned with language variation within and between social groups, its domain is largely that of sociolinguistics.

Language and the way that it is used frequently evokes strong feelings. For example, some teachers and traditionalists propose that language should be taught and studied in a prescriptive manner, with students absorbing and replicating rigid grammatical rules for sentence construction and word formation. Their belief in the desirability of this approach is usually justified in terms of the superiority of the conventional rules for writing and speaking a particular language; thus slang, colloquial speech and certain dialects are derided as being inferior, less accurate and less expressive forms. Unfortunately for them, linguists have found little evidence to support this view; in fact their work demonstrates that virtually all forms of language are fit for the purposes for which they are used. For example, the expressive range and accuracy of the vernacular speech of many black Americans has not been found to be technically inferior in its communicative capacity to the upper-class English used by Ivy League college professors. Linguists recognize that some language variants are perceived socially by some people to be superior or inferior to others, but conclude that there is no intrinsic reason for this – it simply represents the attitudes of the socially dominant groups. Linguistics and sociolinguistics are thus primarily concerned with describing and theorizing about language and language use, not with prescribing preferred forms. As we shall see later in Chapter 5, the debate about 'correct' language use is indeed political but not, perhaps, in quite the way we expect.

The main themes of this book addressed sequentially in the first five chapters are:

- the relationship of language to thought;
- attitudes toward language and attitudes expressed through language;
- the role of language in personal and group identity;

- how we use language in everyday communication;
- the relationship of language to power.

Readers should note that each of the first five chapters is fairly self-contained, so that each may be read separately and in isolation, since the contents largely stand alone, requiring little cross-reference to other chapters – though of course, the cumulative knowledge base that underpins the final two chapters will be compromised. However, if readers wish to skim through the bits of the book that they find most relevant to them, there is a short glossary, which attempts to encapsulate some of the more frequently used and 'difficult' ideas. The main purpose of the glossary is for readers to remind themselves, as they progress through the book, of terms which they are unsure about.

Chapter 1 begins with a consideration of what language is, then outlines the main forms of linguistic variation and begins to explore the complex relationship between language and culture. There is a review of theories about the relationship of language and thought, first from a psychological perspective and then from a linguistic one. These fundamental theories about language are used to consider whether it is possible to think without the concepts that language provides, and also to consider to what extent language reflects or creates our ideas of reality. This chapter introduces the question of whether our thoughts about our world are determined by the pre-existence of the language/s we learn, or whether we have some capacity to think anew. This chapter is inevitably rather theoretical but these apparently esoteric diversions are crucial to the broader purpose of this book, which is concerned with the question of whether we are able to change our ideas about practice, or whether we are stuck with the mind set or world-view that we have learnt. For the casual reader, the first chapter, with its wide-ranging review of theory, might seem a bit daunting: however, I would encourage you to stick with it, on the promise that the subsequent chapters are rather more accessible.

Chapters 2 and 3 illustrate how attitudes to cultural and ethnic differences in language are often based upon unsociological and ahistorical ideas about society. Chapter 2 looks at the relationship between language and attitudes. It examines the growing popularity of English within the world and identifies some of the assumptions that English monoglot speakers may have about their own and other languages. In particular, it begins to examine how language is used to categorize our experiences and perceptions of ourselves and other people. Chapter 3 uses the concept of ethnicity to review the role that language plays in personal and group identity. It reviews two interesting examples of language transformation, where people have used language to differentiate and dissociate themselves from other social groups and thus establish a stronger group identity. The final part of the chapter develops the issue of group and personal identity in situations of social disadvantage and reviews some interesting theoretical ideas about the effects of discrimination upon self and group identity.

Chapter 4 considers some of the research that describes the way in which we actually use language in everyday life. The ideas of the ethnomethodologists, role theorists and communication theorists are reviewed in order to illustrate the extent to which our use of language is constructed and constrained by implicit and informal rules. Chapter 5 begins with the question – what is power? – and in a broad review of the relationship between language and power develops the notion that language use is structured. Using research from microstudies of interpersonal influence and more wide-ranging macrotheories it shows how language and its use can create power, as well as reinforce and conceal its use. The way that we speak, the ideas that we talk about and the particular languages that we choose, or are required to speak in, reveal important information about who has power and who benefits from its exercise.

Chapter 6 critically evaluates current theories in nursing, social work, counselling and communication from the perspective of the knowledge reviewed in the preceding chapters. In many of these theories language is often taken for granted, as if its significance were determined solely by the immediate context of professional/client interaction. Even when writers are sensitive to the cultural context of language use, they often fail to follow through on the implications of their work, the major deficit in most theories is an inadequate conceptualization of key concepts such as culture and power. The chapter concludes that language is a significant factor, that it is not a neutral device and that it should not be subsumed to other factors such as 'race'.

The final chapter attempts to incorporate the most significant elements of the earlier work into an explicit antidiscriminatory approach to health and welfare practice. It considers the raising of awareness about language and identifies the knowledge that is required to develop linguistically-sensitive practice. It provides practical advice on how to establish communication in situations of language difference, and reviews the issue of culturally sensitive practice, the nature of the relationship between the professional and client/patient, and the question of how we might begin to evaluate our practice. Finally, it considers the question of language policies in health and welfare services and offers suggestions as to their content and development.

The book concludes that language alone should not be the sole focus of theory and practice, but that it is a vital element which is frequently ignored or underplayed. My contention is that language use is inevitably a political activity, and while our language and the ideas embodied within it are to some degree presented to us as ready-made, we do have some freedom to change both the meaning and the language itself. We are neither wholly free of, nor wholly determined by our own cultures, professional or personal, or by the structures of power within society and our agencies. The crux of an antidiscriminatory approach to practice is more than an appreciation of cultural and social difference and disadvantage, it is the realization and acceptance of the fact that our own attitudes and behaviour, as well as those of other people, may be unwittingly reinforcing discrimination. This necessitates a proactive approach to the things we do in our work, together with a commitment to resist and challenge the unfair practices which precipitate or contribute to the problems facing many service users. Whether we like it or not, our work is political; we have power that we can use knowingly to benefit others, or we can pretend that we are powerless and abandon them. The aim of this book is to show the crucial role that the language we think and speak with has in constructing our view of the world and how it provides the bridging link to the experience of other people within it.

Finally a word about my own language. I have avoided using masculine pronouns, such as he and his, as generic for both men and women, but where they occur in quotations I have left them as they stand, though they are marked [*sic*]. Consequently, when referring to a single person I have used the slightly clumsy forms her/his and s/he, because these are easily recognized and their meaning generally understood. Similarly, I have avoided the use of collective nouns, such as mankind, that use maleness as the dominant representation for all people. The use of words like black or blind to convey negative connotations about people and things has also been avoided; thus they are only used in their descriptive contexts. The question of how to refer to the people who use our services is a tricky one because of the wide range of intended readership across the health and welfare professions. The conventional terms used within each profession range from client, customer, consumer, patient, case and resident; some terms thus mean more to some professions than others. There is an additional difficulty in that these words are not neutral: they each carry certain connotations about the status of the person who is receiving, in relation to the person who is providing service (see Chapter 5). I have found no easy answer to this problem and have dodged the issue by using the conventional terms when referring to specific examples and using them randomly in all other general references to service users.

Thinking about language

1

Language is a city to the building of which every human being brought a stone.

Emerson, cited in Stevenson, 1974

Conversation is to be thought of as creating a social world just as causality generates a physical one.

Harré, 1983

DEFINING LANGUAGE

These opening quotations are intended to establish the idea firmly in the reader's mind that language is a social creation: it is the result of human action and it can be changed by human action. Emerson emphasizes the collective nature of language use as an activity in which virtually all humans are participants, while Harré stresses the intersubjectivity of our social world, in that it is our use and participation in linguistic activity that shapes our perceptions of the world we live in. For just as cause and effect shapes the scientific perception of the physical world, so speech inevitably shapes our social world.

At the outset the apparently simple question 'what is language?' seems to have a relatively straightforward answer – language is human speech and writing. Unfortunately, this simplicity is deceptive. The question raises many complex issues which anthropologists, philosophers, psychologists and sociologists have tried to tackle, but even linguists are forced to concede that 'Most textbooks on language avoid the problem, preferring to characterize the notion of language rather than define it' (Crystal, 1987). Linguists have developed two approaches to defining language. The first involves attempts to identify universal characteristics possessed by all languages, such as grammar, syntax or classes of words like nouns and verbs (Bloomfield, 1933; Chomsky, 1986). Some attempts at identifying universal characteristics have used the 'butterfly collector' approach, where linguists have studied and collected 'exotic' languages and then attempted to identify the supposedly common features. The second approach is to distinguish language from animal communication, in terms of characteristics such as it being a learned ability as opposed to a genetically transmitted one, or the ability to communicate about things that are not present in the immediate situation (Hockett, 1958). As Witttengenstein observed, his dog might anticipate a juicy bone, but without language could not conceive of next Thursday.

A pragmatic starting point is to regard language as a universal or general category; so that different languages such as Arabic, Chinese, English or French are regarded as varieties or types of language. Each human language, though different, is thus seen to possess certain essential characteristics, such as grammatical rules that determine how words may be ordered or altered and vocabularies that determine the stock of available words. Derrida (1987) suggests that the defining feature of language is its **iterability**, by which he means the fact that it permits the initial utterance of an idea and then allows it to be repeated again over time. The repetition may be by the original speaker or by another person, but in the act of repetition the meaning is always subtly altered, whatever the speaker's intention, because the situation or context is never exactly the same.

DISTINGUISHING SPEECH, SIGNING AND WRITING

It seems, therefore, a simple step to regard speech, signing and writing merely as the technical means by which language is used for communication between people. However, this distinction assigns a rather mechanistic role to writing, which led one writer to conclude: 'Writing is not language... but merely a way of recording language by means of visible marks' (L. Bloomfield, cited in Crystal, 1987). This approach conflicts with the more common view, that a proper language in its purest state is represented by its written form, with the spoken language relegated to secondary status. A surprising number of prominent philosophical and psychological theorists of language, including Chomsky (1968), have followed this line and have consequently developed their ideas about language with little reference to speech at all! Nevertheless, the opposite holds for many anthropologists and linguists whose research has found that while virtually all languages have a spoken form, not all have a written equivalent. Quechua, the language of the Inca people, had no written form, yet they were able to develop and control an impressive state of over 10 million people entirely through an oral culture (Classen, 1993). Consequently, linguists have for many years not only assumed the primacy of speech but tended to equate language entirely with speech.

More recently the view that speech and writing are effectively different languages has gained favour, as detailed research has shown that the 'rules' for speech appear to be quite different from those for writing. The immediate significance of this distinction within linguistics has been to allow the separate study of each type of language without having to reconcile the obvious contradictions between the two. The realization that speech patterns do not wholly follow the rules of sentence construction that determine the patterns of written language has liberated speech analysis and consequently allowed a broader emphasis upon how meaning is established in conversation. Ellis and Beattie (1986) have synthesized a useful table of the characteristic differences between speech and writing (Table 1.1).

Table 1.1 Differences between speech and writing (adapted from Ellis and Beattie, (1986)

Speech	Writing
Normally occurs in the context of shared social activity	Normally occurs in isolation
Immediate feedback from individuals to whom message is directed	Feedback is delayed or non-existent
Development of content is negotiated	Content determined by writer alone
Little revising or editing	Often extensive revision and editing
Syntactically and lexically simple	Syntactically and lexically complex
Message complemented by other communication channels	Single channel only
Brief temporary signal	Enduring signal

Sign languages

This recognition of difference also has implications for understanding other non-verbal means of communication, such as the various forms of sign language. While sign languages, such as British Sign Language, were originally based upon spoken languages, they have become distinct and separate languages, having developed specific rules of use and unique forms of expression which are not always the direct equivalent of words in verbal languages. This differentiation means that users of British and American sign language, both originally based upon English, cannot completely understand each other. Ladd (1991) has noted the irony in the use of American Sign Language in the London production of the successful stage play about deafness, *Children of a Lesser God*, which thoughtlessly disenfranchised the deaf members of the British audience, as most only understood British Sign Language.

Deaf sign languages are widely assumed to be **iconic**; that is, the sign is believed to mimic or act the meaning of a word by an imitative gesture. While most deaf languages do contain some iconic signs, these have typically become highly stylized and are rarely recognizable as such. For example, in British Sign Language, the sign for 'home' is a combination of the original iconic signs for eating and sleeping: 'eat' was made by pursing the fingers to the lips and 'sleep' was made by resting the head, pillow fashion, against one hand; the contemporary sign is simply a single action of pursed fingers twisted at the side of the face (McCrone, 1993). The impetus towards symbolic rather than imitative gestures was also necessary for the development of a fully expressive language, since there are many concepts and words that are not amenable to direct mimicry. The result, of course, is that there is no intrinsic reason why words/signs in one sign language should be similar to those in another.

The idea that sign languages were simply a technical means of communication akin to Morse code or semaphore may have gained currency because the literal translation of a statement in sign language can prove deceptive. It may create the impression that the language is somewhat simplistic and ungrammatical; whereas the original statement may have been perfectly acceptable and comprehensible to another sign user. Sign languages typically do not sign sequences of individual words, which is slow and unwieldy, but communicate whole phrases or concepts; this enhances rapid communication and thus sign languages have established distinctive vocabularies of meaning that are as rich and subtle as those of spoken languages. The unfavourable comparisons arising from literal translation are also based upon an assumed notion of perfect spoken English as the norm for spoken conversation; however, linguists have shown that this ideal form of standard English with Received Pronunciation, that is, the classic BBC style, is rarely used outside formal contexts such as news broadcasting and speeches. Ordinary vernacular speech, when represented in writing, is full of half-finished statements, unanswered questions, hesitations and *non sequiturs*; hence the unfavourable comparison arises, in part, from a misunderstanding of how sign languages operate and from the use of an idealized criterion for the comparison.

LINGUISTIC VARIATION

The most obvious form of variation is that evidenced by the tremendous number of different languages. Crystal (1987) notes that estimates vary from between 3000 and 10 000 languages, which reflects differences in defining what counts as a language and also the absence of sufficient reliable survey information about spoken languages. However, linguistic variation is not confined solely to types of language or the means of communicating them. There are significant distinctions of nationality, dialect and accent, a dialect, for example, being usually thought of as a variety of a given language rather than a separate type (Romaine, 1994). The 'common-sense' linguistic criterion for assessing whether one language is different from another is based upon the idea of intelligibility; thus if two speakers cannot understand each other, they are assumed to be speaking different languages, that is, they are mutually unintelligible. Unfortunately, this approach does not adequately capture the reality of how people use and view their languages. While there are relatively small differences between Serbian and Croatian, or Hindi and Urdu, or Danish and Swedish, for the native speakers of each of these the perceived differences may be crucially important. As we shall see in Chapter 4, the significance lies in the assertion of group identity.

While English may appear to be a language that many of us share, the variations of dialect may be so great as to impair communication between different dialect groups. The well known statement that Britain and the United States are two nations separated by a common language indicates the general recognition of significant differences in dialect, accent, grammar and vocabulary; but the variation in these features of language may be so great as to render mutually incomprehensible conversation between members of different dialect groups. During the Second World War well-educated, middle-class Jamaican volunteers, who travelled by boat from the West Indies to Scotland and then by train to England, enquired in Newcastle what language the local people were speaking. Their puzzlement and curiosity arose from the prevalent vernacular 'geordie' dialect and accent, which they found incomprehensible, it was unrecognizable to them as a form of English (snippet of oral history heard on Radio 4, source unknown).

British-born speakers of English who use words such as 'rubber' and 'faggot', for 'eraser' and 'meatball', may be embarrassed to find that, to North Americans, these words respectively mean 'condom' and 'male homosexual'. Their confusion may be compounded when a multitude of other, apparently universal terms, like 'auger', 'pavement', 'escalator' and 'common-law husband', are also greeted with blank looks. Similarly, common US words and phrases, such as 'duplex', 'boxscore', 'crosswalk' and 'realtor', may leave the British speaker of English mystified (Bryson, 1990). Misunderstandings can also be generated by a failure to appreciate how much the meaning of words and sentences depends upon shared knowledge and an understanding of the idiomatic and formulaic 'rules' for using a language. Phrases such as 'break a leg' (theatre-speak for 'good luck'), 'how are you?' and 'have a nice day' are not literal but ritualistic expressions. You are not expected to literally injure yourself, or recite precisely and in detail exactly how you are feeling. In fact, if you do so, others will quickly become exasperated with your misunderstanding of the informal conversational gambit they are using (Garfinkel, 1967). Gumperz (1982b) has noted that this type of misunderstanding is most problematic for people 'who ostensibly speak the same language but come from different social or regional backgrounds. Since they assume that they understand each other, they are less likely to question interpretations'.

In addition to the variations of dialect and accent, linguists have made many other analytical distinctions; Table 1.2, adapted from Crystal (1987), represents one model of these, with three basic aspects – meaning, grammar, and medium of transmission. In turn, these are further subdivided.

Table 1.2 Analysis of language (adapted from Crystal, 1987)

Meaning (semantics)	{	Lexicon (vocabulary)
		Discourse (broad patterns of meanings)
Grammar	{	Syntax (rules for the organization of words)
		Morphology (word structure)
Medium of transmission	{	Phonetics (pronunciation)
		Phonology (patterns of sound)

Despite these technical distinctions, for workers in the human services, an appreciation of the importance of language use and variation does not have to be based upon detailed knowledge of all of these differences, but upon understanding the fundamental notion that most language variation is structured, not random or accidental. By this I mean that most differences in and between languages are not incidental variations that arise from individuals choosing and using language as they please, but are regular features, which represent important differences in such things as attitude, identity, power and status. The following chapters explore some of the implications of these structured differences.

Language and culture

Culture in the sociological sense refers to the shared understandings, perceptions and ways of living that are common within a society or social group. Argyle (1983) provides a typical definition of culture, which he takes to include 'their whole way of life – their language, ways of perceiving, categorizing and thinking about the world, forms of non-verbal communication and social interaction, rules and conventions about behaviour, moral values and ideals, technology and material culture, art, science, literature and history'. This broad concept of culture explicitly recognizes the interlinking of ideas and action, and stands in contradiction to the common or lay view of culture as essentially high literature and the fine arts such as painting, sculpture and so on. Nevertheless, Said (1993) has elegantly stated the perils of assuming that a narrow culture of 'the arts' is somehow transcendent and divorced from the social milieu from which it originates and the social reality which it creates and sustains. Said's point is that art is a human creation, created by particular people living in particular societies at particular periods in history. Thus the broader notion of culture, as will become apparent from the ideas and theories discussed later in this book, is conceptualized, represented and reiterated through language. Carter and Aitchison (1986) summarize this view: 'The character and vitality of a culture is to a large extent language dependent. Language helps to preserve traditions, shapes modes of perception and profoundly influences patterns of social intercourse and behaviour.' Therefore, acceptance of this broader sociological conception of culture is a prerequisite for developing an understanding of the intricate and complex relationship of language to culture. A relationship is made more complex by the twofold role of language as 'more than a means of expression but also the product and carrier of social culture' (Pugh, 1992). Words do not simply represent things but embody the modes of thinking that lead to their creation, selection and use. The meaning and use of language signifies the relative value of particular people, objects and actions within particular societies. Describing a person as a 'service-user', 'patient', 'client' or 'customer' indicates the professional worker's more or less explicit view of the nature of the relationship with the recipients of the service.

In Western industrialized societies the tremendous emphasis upon visual representations of culture through imagery and writing has made most of us unaware of the extent to which our relationship to our world is mediated primarily through vision and secondarily through sound. The hierarchical ordering of the senses – vision, sound, smell, taste and touch – predates Aristotle's authoritative ranking and remains dominant in Western societies (Vinge, 1975). Classen (1993) reminds us that this has not always been the case and should not be assumed to be a universal phenomenon. Classen describes how different cultures have alternative rankings and conceptually order their world view according to these. In Mexico the Tzotzil people use a thermal symbolism to make sense of their world, people and things being understood in terms of their temperature. The compass point east, being the direction of the rising sun, is known as 'lok' eb k' ak' al', the emerging heat; while the west is called 'maleb k' ak' al', meaning the waning heat.

> Everything in the universe is thought to contain a different quantity of heat... men are believed to possess more heat than women. Making women symbolically cold by contrast.... Newborns... are bathed in warm water, censed, wrapped in blankets and ritually presented with 'hot' chilli peppers, in order to keep them warm until they have acquired enough heat to survive on their own.
>
> *Classen, 1993*

In a similar manner the Ongee people of Little Andaman Island order their world by smell. Odour is fundamental to personal identity; thus when Ongee people wish to refer to themselves as individuals, the speaker touches her/his nose. The significance of smell as an ordering concept is not wholly absent in Western societies, as the power of insults concerning offensive odours indicates. These attributions, like variations in languages, are not random, the negative attribution of an unpleasant odour to women in menstruation having a long history and indicating the nature of male attitudes towards women and their sexuality. The common stereotype of 'smelly foreigners' also reflects a fear of difference, of the outsider, and may similarly be used to justify discriminatory actions. Ironically, most Westerners are unaware that their characteristic odour, to many people from countries where relatively few animal products are eaten, is that of rancid fat!

Confusion and misunderstanding may arise from differences such as dialect, accent and vocabulary but can also be generated by differences in the world-view or conceptual structure of understanding embodied within different languages. The language used by a doctor in consultation with a patient may signify superior knowledge, status and power, but the interaction, far from elic-iting an accurate summary of presenting symptoms, may actually lead to confu-sion and misdiagnosis. Ely and Denney (1987) noted the confusion that arose when an Asian woman was asked by a psychiatrist 'how do you feel in your-self?' Her response, to the effect that her family was fine, was interpreted as evidence of her mental distress, whereas its meaning for her lay in the social conception of herself not as a solitary psyche but as a mother, wife and daugh-ter, that is, in relation to the health and well-being of the significant people in her life. They comment that 'many Asian patients may be less concerned with what is going on in their own heads, [and more concerned] with their roles and positions in society.... If you can fulfil your obligations and your role you are well; if you cannot you are ill.'

Thus, the individualistic conception of self, predominant in Western society and represented in this instance through the phrase 'in yourself', is not univer-sally shared by all people. Even the assumption that patients share the same understanding of common medical terms may be misguided. Boyle (1975) in a study of English monoglot doctors and patients, found that while all doctors agreed that 'heartburn' referred to 'a burning sensation behind the breastbone', 8% of patients thought it meant 'passage of wind through the mouth', while a further 4.5% thought it referred to 'excess saliva'! The risks arising from such ambiguity are obvious.

LANGUAGE AND THOUGHT – PSYCHOLOGICAL APPROACHES

Perhaps the most interesting and important debate is that surrounding the rela-tionship of language and consciousness, that is, the question of whether language provides the conceptual structures we use for perceiving the external world. Within psychology, this issue has centred on whether thought precedes language, or whether language is a necessary prerequisite of conscious thought. Thus Western psychologists have been less concerned with the extent to which language itself may be determined by social factors, and have preferred to focus on how individuals learn and acquire language (Greene, 1975). For many years there were basically two positions on language learning: the behaviourist view, led by Skinner (1957) and Watson (1924), and the cognitive view, epitomized by Chomsky (1968, 1986) and Piaget (1959).

The behaviourist position

The behaviourists (Skinner, 1957; Watson, 1924), in their quest for scientific rigour, largely discounted or denied the existence of internal concepts such as consciousness and cognition, because their existence could not be validated by direct observation. They believed that children learnt language through classical and operant conditioning, that is, through the repetitive mechanisms of stimulus/action and response. Their view was that social conditioning alone accounted for the development of the full repertoire of language, without any need to refer to intervening processes. The behaviourist tradition, therefore, is unable to directly answer the question of the precedence of thought versus language, because it essentially denies one of the basic concepts – thought. Arguably, the implication of their stance with regard to the primacy of language and thought is that language is the predominant factor and that it is a relativistic one at that. Watson stated that 'the behaviourist advances the view that what psychologists have hitherto called thought is nothing but talking to ourselves' (cited in McCrone, 1993). Although behaviourists do not accept the validity of such concepts as perception, it is clear that, if language learning is conditioned, then it follows that children can only learn the language of the situations that they experience. Even if the original proponents of behaviourism were unable to countenance such abstract intervening mechanisms of perception, the potential for different ideas or conceptual structures of the world is nevertheless present. Difference may arise simply from the different locations of language users within the social and physical world. Most behaviourist approaches are subject to the general criticism that they portray a human actor who is almost totally determined by her/his environment. A more specific criticism, is that there is no account of how the language and its meanings are established in the first place. Admittedly this is not a problem for strict behaviourists but few behavioural psychologists today would accept the absence of subjective concepts, such as meaning, in understanding our use of language.

The cognitive position

The cognitive tradition within psychology largely accepts the relevance of the behaviourist account in explaining the processes of simple learning, but is critical of the omission of intervening processes of cognition. While the behaviourists saw children as a blank page upon which language was written, the cognitivists embraced developmental models of language learning which implied either innate predispositions to learn language (Chomsky, 1968), or at least, neuropsychological limits to the development of language and thinking at particular ages and stages (Piaget, 1959). Chomsky contends that all humans have an innate capacity for language learning, in other words, to use an electrical analogy, they are pre-wired with a **language acquisition device**. The basis of Chomsky's argument is that the behaviourist account does not adequately explain how it is possible for children to produce new sentences and manipulate word meanings without some appreciation of the complex and extensive rules of language, an appreciation of what he calls the **deep structure** of language. Explicit in this approach is the premise that all languages have universal underlying principles that govern their use, and therefore all children have the potential to learn any language. Again the question of the precedence of thought versus language is not clearly answered. The proposition that there is an inherent capacity to learn language implies that language is dominant, at least in terms of its deep structure and broad principles, but this says little about the question of content.

Chomsky's position also has its problems. First, his analysis of the universal features of language concentrates almost exclusively upon the formal structures of sentences and thus tends to ignore the reality of how people actually speak to each other (Akinasso, 1982). As noted earlier, normal vernacular speech has many unfinished, incomplete sentences and single word utterances that clearly mean something to the participants but simply cannot be accounted for by the abstract rules Chomsky posits. Second, the emphasis upon innate abilities arguably overemphasizes the genetic inheritance of humans and underplays the social factors which influence language learning and use. In doing this Chomsky is repeating the error of omission made by many linguists, as Cameron (1992) comments: 'Even grammatical patterns that appear to be social and political in their motivation – like pronoun usage in English – have been explained by mainstream linguists in completely non-social terms.'

Piaget differs in his view of precedence. His maturational model of child development contends that thought precedes the meaningful use of language. Piaget took the view that external events and actions are learned (memorized/internalized) and then words are attached to them. He believed that children were innately determined to the extent that they could only demonstrate certain forms of thought at particular ages and stages. His model has been wittily described by McCrone (1993) as a horticultural one, in which children and their various mental abilities are all present in the beginning seed, and that the role of good parents and teachers is therefore to nurture the pre-existing potential that lies within them. Piaget concedes that children can appear to learn languages before the optimum stages of development, in the sense that they can be taught words, but that this has no more developmental significance than words memorized by a parrot (Dobson *et al.*, 1982)! In this account, to learn a language involves the development of an internal memory of meaningful events and ideas experienced, so for language to mean anything it has to be preceded by thought.

In contradiction to this view, Vygotsky (1962), from his observations of what Piaget termed the **egocentric** speech of young children – that is, the language spoken aloud but not apparently intended or aimed at anyone, disagreed with his conclusion that this was meaningless babble. Vygotsky took the view that this form of speech was a halfway house between speech aimed at others and silent inner thoughts. He proposed that thought becomes initially structured during the silent phases of language learning; in other words that the words learned provided the conceptual frameworks of meaning. This inner thought is initially slow and elementary but gains in speed and sophistication as the child develops this inner voice through the learning of language. As the child matures the inner voice is less apparent in overtly self-directed speech, such as the descriptions of things and the instructions for action which children speak to themselves, but nevertheless continues as it becomes the silent inner voice of the mind. Ironically, after reading some of Vygotsky's work, Piaget later amended his view of egocentric speech and conceded its necessity, but he failed to realize the full implications of Vygotsky's broad theory, an approach which ultimately rejects the idea of an innate pre-programmed pattern for the development of thought (McCrone, 1993).

LANGUAGE AND THOUGHT – THE LINGUISTIC TRADITION

Within linguistics the modern formulation of the question of whether language determines thought has developed from the work of Saussure, whose ideas were first published after his death in 1916 under the title *Cours de linguistique generale/Course in General Linguistics* (1974). Saussure is acknowledged as the founder of **semiology/semiotics**, an approach in which language is but one aspect of the study of the role of signs and signals in human communication. One of his main tenets was the proposal that no word or other symbol (signifier) had any intrinsic link with the thing that it represented (significd). Thus, spoken words were sounds which symbolized other things, and writing too was a symbolic system of marks that represented and conveyed meaning about other things. Unlike previous linguistic studies, his focus was not concerned with how a language changed over time (dinchronic analysis), but with how it could be analysed at a given point (synchronic analysis). As we shall see later, this recognition of the arbitrary nature of the relationship between actual words and the things they represented was a crucial step in considering the relationship between languages and the world they purport to represent. His method of analysis attempted to distinguish the component parts of formal language and then describe their functions in relation to each other. Anthropologists like Boas and Levi-Strauss enthusiastically adopted and developed this synchronic method, which they termed structuralism, to study spoken language and sign systems among people who had no written history and whose language could therefore only be studied contemporaneously. The American anthropologist Sapir (1929), in his studies of North American Indian languages, quickly recognized that there was considerable variation in the view of the world espoused by the speakers of different languages. 'The worlds in which different societies live are distinct worlds, not merely the same world with different labels attached.'

This of course raised questions regarding the significance of such differences and the role of language in creating and sustaining such variation.

Sapir, together with Benjamin Whorf (1976), in the eponymous Sapir–Whorf hypothesis, then developed a theory of language which posited that the speaker's language acted as a series of categories through which the world was perceived; that each language provides a grid through which the external world is conceptualized and experienced. Thus different languages potentially provide different grids or frameworks through which the person and the group experience their world; hence the language learnt and used by a person shapes her/his perception of the world and events within it. Thus the adult identification of personal feelings such as nostalgia or melancholia, represents a shaping of perception from the earliest distinctions that will have been learnt in childhood, such as of being happy or sad. Their hypothesis tackled the two central issues about language and thought. The first, was the question of **linguistic determinism**, which considered whether feelings and thoughts preceded language, in the sense that they were experienced and then named, as opposed to the notion that they were conditioned and shaped by the learning of language. For Sapir and Whorf the answer was unequivocal: language precedes thought and therefore shapes or constructs it. The second question was about the issue of **linguistic relativism**, that is, the extent to which all languages describe or construct the same world-view, as opposed to the idea that words and the concepts embodied within them are unique to each language. Their conclusion, that languages did not describe a universal reality, followed logically from the acceptance of linguistic determinism and furthermore appeared to fit the facts gained from their field research. Thus the world-views established within different languages could have unique features and hence were relative conceptions of reality, established and maintained uniquely within each language.

For linguists acceptance of the thesis of linguistic relativity meant that there was no exact or necessary correspondence between different languages, and for anthropologists it raised a further problem about whether it was possible to understand and appreciate the different world-views of different people. For both disciplines the answer was the same: no understanding was possible without competence within the respective language, and even with this, comprehension of the differences might only be partial. Sapir contended that it was almost impossible for observers to appreciate those behaviours of other people which appeared similar to established patterns within their own, without imposing these external meanings upon them.

Sapir and Whorf's individual ideas are often conflated as if they were identical in all respects but, as Williams (1992) has noted, there are important differences in their positions with regard to the formation of language and their models of the external world. 'Sapir saw language as formed in the social world and suggests that it is not until after it is formed that it operates to shape a world view.... In contrast, Whorf... saw the external world as merely chaotic without the intervention of the linguistic system.'

The distinction is between Sapir's view, that it is not possible to fully appreciate or know the external world until one has learnt the social language to describe it, and Whorf's, that the chaotic external world impresses itself upon the person regardless of language, but that it is language which creates order in the mind of the person perceiving the world. A fuller discussion of their differences is provided in Williams (1992).

Before addressing some of the main criticisms of their hypothesis, it is important to note that, while strong versions of linguistic determinism such as that presented by Spender (1980) are open to obvious criticism, such overly deterministic accounts need not be taken as representative of the Whorfian tradition generally, nor do they diminish the potential value of the ideas. For example, while Spender's account – of how the 'man-made' rules of meaning embodied within language operate to maintain the subjugation of women within a patriarchal world – has been a great stimulus to the development of a feminist perspective in linguistics, her theoretical position is flawed. Cameron (1992) acknowledges the accuracy of many of Spender's observations, but also demonstrates the theoretical inconsistencies in her approach. Nevertheless, as we shall see in the discussion of Cameron's critique in Chapter 4, the problems that beset Spender's rendition of linguistic determinism are not necessarily inherent in weaker versions of the Sapir–Whorf hypothesis.

Fishman (1980) has noted the main points of criticism of the Whorfian approach, which are that:

- it does not offer a convincing explanation of the origin of language structures;
- it underplays the extent to which change can occur;
- the explanation tends to operate in one direction, that is, where language is perceived as the cause of events in thought and in the external world, whereas there may be an interplay between them or in some instances the causes lie elsewhere.

It is a contentious issue as to how variation occurs in the first place; it is easier to understand its transmission than to explain the sources of variation. Some writers, such as Spender, are quite explicit about an underpinning theory of power which seeks to explain why some people are able to change language and others are not. However, the Sapir–Whorf hypothesis is frequently cited in support of more general accounts of social differentiation without any underpinning theory of power or influence. An equally damaging criticism is that while seeking to explain language variation, the proponents of the hypothesis have exaggerated the consistency and congruence of world-views held **within** a language group, and correspondingly, have exaggerated the differences **between** languages, and thus have understated the similarities between languages and world-views. While linguistic determinism may persuasively account for the negative attributions attached to the colour black in racist societies, and so make comprehensible the social processes of stigmatization. It is arguable that the widespread symbolic distinction made in many languages between the colours black and white, may derive originally from the physical reality of night and day and the accompanying fear of darkness, predators and enemies. The implication is that while some words, including black in its modern meanings, are clearly socially constructed by human action, there are many others whose concept, if not form, arises directly from the external world. Words for body parts, animals, water, trees, earth and sky are present in virtually every language in the world and provide examples of how the relationship of language to the external world must, to some extent, be understood as a two-way process. However, the relationship between the meanings of words and their subjects is by no means a simple one, and it is important to recognize that it may change. For example, the modern connotations of the words black and white derive from the historical European exploration of the other continents. White colonists characterized the different 'races' they encountered as either black or white, and in doing so attached the pre-existing symbolic meanings of black and white to them (Jordan, 1974). This derogation of the category 'black' then served as a convenient rationale for the killing and exploitation of such people.

In contradiction to the theory of linguistic determinism one could conceive of a one-way relationship in the other direction. Instead of language determining thought and the world-view, that is, from the person-with-language to the external world; the pattern of dominance could flow in the opposite direction, that is, from the external world to the person. Such an approach presumes the predominance of the external world and conceives of language as being a reactive response to this world. Thus language and the concepts embodied within particular words could be seen as direct representations of this external reality. Trudgill (1983) describes how this process may operate from both the physical and the social environment. The fact that the Inuit (Eskimo) have many words for snow while the Bedouin have an extensive vocabulary for camels reflects the relative importance of these things in their lives, and their presence in the respective languages is derived directly from the external physical world. Similarly, the external social world of particular groups and individuals could be reflected in the conceptual vocabularies that describe them. Thus, relationships such as family lines of descent or patterns of authority, which are often specific and relatively unique to particular societies, would be indicated by the language developed to describe them. For example, the Turkish word *yenge*, meaning 'wife of a friend', has no direct equivalent in English because we do not recognize or mark this relationship in the same way (Caine, 1993). As we shall see later, besides the contested question of whether the physical world influences language in this way, the extrapolation of the argument into the social world is indeed a contentious point, especially with regard to the issue of cause and effect.

However, according to this outward-in, world-determined view of language, changes in the social and physical world are consequently reflected by changes in language. Thus, within the last 30 years the changing position and perception of black people is marked by the changing use of language, from 'negro' to 'coloured' to 'black' and most recently in North America, to the phrase 'people of colour'. Similarly, the feminist critique of existing social relations has problematized the unthinking use of masculine nouns and pronouns such as 'chairman', 'he' and 'his' as if they were general categories for all people, by demonstrating how such **androcentric** assumptions reinforce patterns of dominance and disadvantage (Spender, 1980; Cameron, 1992). However, the major weakness of this world-determining approach is that, while attributing changes in language to changes in the external world, it leaves unanswered the question of how this changes in the first place. Whereas in the language-determined approach language variation is due to differentiation in the acquired conceptual structure inherent in different languages, in the world-determined approach, where the relationship is reversed and the world shapes the language, linguistic variation derives from different social and geographical locations within the world.

In philosophy the metaphysical question of the extent to which actors create or are created by the world has long been the subject of study and debate. Within the social sciences there has been a matching concern with determinism and individual choice in explanations of society (Mannheim, 1959; Wrong, 1961; Giddens, 1984). This has been most apparent within the sociology of deviance, where several approaches have acknowledged both the historical/structural and the personal/interactionist elements in their explanations, and thus attempted to resolve the apparent conflict (Taylor, Walton and Young, 1973; Dallos and Sapsford, 1981). From a psychological perspective one of the most interesting attempts to restructure the question has come from John McCrone (1993). He has forcefully argued that the basic problem with the existing nature/nurture debates about human thought and language, arises not solely from the mutually exclusive nature of such either/or propositions but from a basic misconception about language and the human mind.

As we have seen earlier, most earlier approaches to the subject proposed either an innate capacity to develop language or some model of social learning; McCrone believes that both approaches are simply missing the point and have misread the existing evidence, which supports a different model. He argues that the dominant tradition in Western thought has been one that contrasts rationality with irrationality: rationality being all of the operations of the mind that are open to conscious and selective manipulation, and the irrational being represented by all of the emotional states and processes that are not. Freud's ideas on the primitive urges of the id, the unconscious processes and memories of the mind are but one example of how the irrational has been used to 'explain' the apparent abberations and conflicts of human behaviour and thought. For McCrone, however, the explanation of how we think and operate is much simpler: he argues that the human brain is not sufficiently different in its size or qualities to explain why we are so different from other animals. It is the conscious and extensive use of language, he argues, that differentiates us from animals and it is language that allows a better use of the capacities of our brains. Using the analogy of a computer, he argues that the basic physiology and chemistry of our brains resemble a computer that comes with simple pre-programmed routines, such as limited memory and some capacity for intentional activity, but that it is language which acts as a super-programme that enables a fuller use of its potential capacity.

One difficulty we may have in accepting McCrone's idea is that it relegates language, and by implication the thoughts we are able to think with it, to the level of more mundane inventions like the wheel. But just as the wheel when used in a bicycle is able to multiply our physical efforts and allow us to travel further and faster than we ever could without it, so language does the same for the development of our thinking. McCrone accepts the proposition that there are optimal periods in a child's early years for language acquisition. Using examples drawn from the successive failures in educating so called 'wild' or feral children, together with evidence from the language learning difficulties faced by deaf children, he argues when language learning is not available during the optimal period and so does not occur, or whenever it is obstructed for whatever reason, the outcome is always the same – a limited ability to think and reason. Failure to successfully achieve competence in some form of symbolic language, whether speech- or sign-based, within the critical period, leaves the brain with the capacity, but not the program that optimizes its use. Thus the suppression of sign language for many years in the education of severely deaf people resulted in the denial of the one language that could enhance their progress, since their capacity in oral languages was always compromised by their hearing impairment (see reference to Ladd in Chapter 2).

Drawing extensively upon the ideas of Vygotsky (1962, Van der Veer and Valsiner, 1991) and the work of Luria (1973, Cole and Cole, 1979), McCrone believes that the development of an inner language of representation, which is normally learnt from the spoken language that surrounds a child, is an absolute prerequisite for effective thinking. In deaf children a symbolic language of signs can fulfil exactly the same functions. This inner language is not merely a preoperative stage of language learning in children, it is the basis of virtually all subsequent thought in adults. McCrone believes that some thoughts precede the learning of language, but that most of what we recognize as cognitive processes are either enhanced immeasurably by language, as in the case of conscious recollection of memory, or actually created by it, as in the instance of reasoning and logic. For McCrone, there is therefore no doubt about the issue of precedence: language precedes most of the thinking processes which are distinctively human, thus in the most fundamental sense thought is shaped by language. Furthermore, different languages, to the extent that they represent significant differences in culture, do inculcate differing world views and even different thinking patterns, which at a broader level indicates the relative nature of all languages.

The obvious question is whether, within linguistics, a similar resolution of the questions of linguistic determinism and linguistic relativity can also be achieved. For example, are the two positions represented by the Sapir–Whorf hypothesis and the world-determined position necessarily mutually exclusive? Stated baldly they appear to be mutually contradictory positions, but if the linguistic determinist approach is not stated in its strongest form and if the world-determined approach accepts that people may consciously act upon the external world, then some reconciliation of the two positions may be attempted. For if people can actively change the social and physical world they live in, then it is apparent that language, far from being a neutral representation of external reality, is to some degree subject to human agency (action plus intention). So while Trudgill (1983) suggests that 'any strong form of the Sapir–Whorf hypothesis – say, that thought is actually constrained by language – cannot be accepted', in conceding that 'habitual thought is to a certain extent conditioned by language', he accepts the likelihood that there is a two-way relationship. Cameron (1992), in her outstanding review of the implications of linguistic theories for feminism, comes to a similar conclusion:

> I agree with those Whorfians and semiologists who suggest that human beings are creatures of culture, their personalities, desires, ways of behaving and understanding constructed by the societies into which they are born, the traditions they inherit. I agree also that not all of the forces shaping us, perhaps not even most of them are easily available to our conscious introspection....Yet I cannot accept a theory in which human beings are denied all agency and all capacity for self-reflection.
>
> *Cameron, 1992*

As Cameron's last sentence indicates, there is no consensus as to how far these processes operate in either direction, nor even agreement as to their accessibility or significance, but there is an acceptance of both possibilities. McCrone (1993) notes that psychological explanations of language and thought have been bedevilled by a philosophy of strict reductionism, which has led to a predominant focus upon the biological aspects of the brain and has avoided the equally important sociology of language and culture: 'We need to head in one direction to explain the mind's hardware, but quite the opposite direction to explain its software'. The academic discipline of linguistics in its own quest for scientific credibility may also be accused of such monodirectional thinking.

CONCLUSION

By now it should be apparent that language is indeed a complex subject, for as soon as we begin to explore what it is, we are faced with some fundamental questions about human psychology and society – what does language represent when we use it and what is the role of language in our relationship to society? If language is a social creation, do we play any part in its creation? Historically, many sociological and psychological theories have presented a picture of the social world in which on one hand we have society and on the other the individual (Burkitt, 1991). Within this dualism, they have presented differing accounts of the nature of the relationship between the two entities. At one end of a continuum are deterministic theories like Parsons' (1937, 1960), which propose that individuals from birth are socialized into prescribed behavioural norms and social roles and, with the exception of criminals and 'deviants', behave accordingly. At the other end, we have accounts that stress the agency of the individual, that is, the capacity to act freely and exercise self-determination (Rogers, 1951, 1967). Between these two poles are a range of theories which, more or less explicitly, acknowledge that individuals are constrained by the power of others, but do not assume the inevitability of its exercise or success. They range from the historical determinism of Marx (1975), who portrays a society in which there are strong social forces whose success, though not inevitable, is difficult to resist; to the various interactionist approaches which allow a greater potential for human agency (action plus intention). Garfinkel (1967), for example, argued persuasively that individuals could think for themselves and did not have to accept the ideas about society and themselves that others might attempt to impose; individuals were not 'judgemental and cultural dopes' (Heritage, 1984). Furthermore, social norms and roles were not static and solid but were continually being constructed and reconstructed as people went about their daily business.

Latterly, the social constructionist theory of Berger and Luckman (1967), which identified the crucial role that language played in establishing our ideas of ourselves and of society, has influenced the work of Shotter (1984, 1993) and Giddens (1984), both of whom reject the dualistic model of society. Society is not perceived as some reified concrete object which is 'out there', beyond us; social structures such as class, gender and race are the product of our thoughts and actions and those of other people. Therefore, they are not real objects, only real ideas, in the sense that they have real consequences when people base their actions upon them. Language is central to this, because it is language which provides the available ideas and categories with which we think and upon which we act, and that acts as the bridge between ourselves and others.

The major theme of this book, therefore, is an examination of the significance of language in terms of social attitudes, personal and group identity, professional interaction and power. Each of the four following chapters will explore these aspects of language variation and begin to identify their implications for our work; they will draw upon a number of academic disciplines to illustrate the complex web of linguistic factors which influence the social interaction and subjective experience of health and welfare workers, and their clients.

2

Attitudes and language

My soul frets in the shadow of his language.

Joyce, 1964

INTRODUCTION

Chapter 1 reviewed theories about the relationship between language and thought, and indicated how language embodies ideas about the world and provides conceptual structures for understanding it. Choosing which words to use is not a neutral nor a purely technical exercise, because the particular meanings we attach to words reveal the underlying values and attitudes about the things we write and talk about. This chapter explores the relationship between attitudes and language. It makes a distinction between attitudes expressed through the use of language, that is, attitudes to things, people, ideas and so on; and attitudes towards language, that is, attitudes about English, and about multi- and bilingualism in particular.

The concept of attitude is one of the building blocks of social psychology, but despite its widespread use there is no complete agreement about what an attitude is. Baker (1992), for example, offers the following working definition: 'Attitudes are a convenient and efficient way of explaining consistent patterns in behaviour. Attitudes often manage to summarize, explain and predict behaviour.' Many social psychologists think of an attitude as being an internal or latent construct that exists within a person's mind, which cannot be directly observed but may be inferred from their behaviour. However, this approach does not adequately capture the sense in which attitudes imply judgement or evaluation. Ajzen (1988) captures this aspect succinctly, when stating that an attitude is 'a disposition to respond favourably or unfavourably to an object, person, institution or event'.

In order to appreciate the relationship between language and attitudes, it is useful to make the distinction noted in the first paragraph. First, there is the way in which language is used to express attitudes. In this case, the actual language type is not itself the subject of the attitude, since the language is being used to carry or signify a person's attitude towards some other person or object; thus their choice of words and language indicates their judgement or evaluation. Changes in attitudes are therefore revealed by changes in the language used to describe or evaluate other people, objects and ideas. There are a number of ways in which this occurs. For example, during the last 20 years, the widespread use of the word 'gay' indicates a shift in public attitudes toward homosexuality, which is signalled by the use of this word in preference to other more judgemental terms. This change in language is particularly interesting because homosexual people themselves decided to redefine the meaning of the word. Another way in which language signals attitudinal change is through the significance attached to particular words. For example, the greater tolerance of some previously unacceptable swear words is marked by their more frequent public use.

The second part of the distinction refers to the attitudes that people hold toward their own language type and their attitudes towards other types. In some instances these attitudes are explicit. For example, in the Basque and Catalan areas of northern Spain it is considered offensive to speak Castilian (Spanish) in some situations, because it symbolically represents the unwanted intrusion of central government power. Negative attitudes towards minority languages can have disastrous effects upon the linguistic minority. In the early years of this century, in both Wales and France it was thought to be a sign of poor education to speak Welsh or Occitan (or any of the other older languages of France), rather than English or French. Thus many people were discouraged, if not prohibited, from speaking their native language. In other cases, the attitudes may be less obvious; they may rest upon implicit assumptions which can be especially damaging for minority languages. Ladd (1991) has described how people who use British Sign Language have typically been viewed as a handicapped group rather than as a linguistic minority. This is because the linguistic norm for Britain has been assumed to be English, and any variation from it, such as sign language or bilingualism, is thus perceived as being abnormal. The consequences of these implicit assumptions and explicit attitudes toward linguistic variation can be extremely damaging. The historical suppression of signing, through the emphasis upon oral language and lip reading, together with the exclusion of deaf teachers from deaf education, severely disadvantaged many deaf people. This second aspect of the distinction, of attitudes to language, is developed next, while the discussion of attitudes **in** language is developed afterwards.

ATTITUDES TO LANGUAGE

The popularity of English

This section examines some of the assumptions held about languages; it begins with a review of those held about English by many first-language English speakers. The increasing dominance of their language throughout the world makes it difficult for them to appreciate the significance of other languages to other people. For example, they may attribute this increasing influence to the linguistic superiority of English and thus assume the technical inferiority of other languages, believing them to be less useful. Such assumptions are widely held and may, in some circumstances, constitute an ideology of language. Ideologies are sets of beliefs, which may be inaccurate fictions but which nevertheless have important consequences, for they may preserve and legitimize existing social structures and so disguise or justify the actions of those who wield power (Habermas, 1970; Mannheim, 1959; McLellan, 1995; Hodge and Kress, 1993). For many English speakers, the ideology of their own language presents and presupposes a particular view of the world, which contains beliefs and assumptions about English *vis-à-vis* other languages.

These beliefs promote an uncritically positive attitude towards English and a correspondingly negative one towards most other languages. There is a fuller discussion of ideology in Chapter 5.

To be an English monoglot speaker is to grow up, be educated, employed and entertained in a language which is rapidly becoming the dominant language of the industrialized world. Ironically, despite the efforts of the Académie Française, English has become the *lingua franca* of medicine, science, computing, air travel and increasingly of business too. In France, the Pasteur Institute no longer publishes its papers in French but English. When Volkswagen built a new factory in China the daily language for communication between local employees and the German managers was English (Bryson, 1990). English monoglots live in a world where their language is now spoken by over 350 million people and is used as an official or semi-official language in over 60 countries, a world where the domains of language extend from travel, entertainment and sport into the formal settings of diplomacy, education, research and business (Crystal, 1987). Monoglot English speakers have come to expect interviews with politicians, survivors of catastrophes, soldiers and sports figures from around the world in English. Their world view is rapidly becoming one in which they expect that events will be accessible to them in their own language; while they may have lost a political empire, they assume that they have gained a linguistic one. Little do they realize that, as English becomes more widely used, it is less and less their property: control of its development and of its meanings increasingly lies with other people.

The growing popularity of English is buttressed by an awareness of its attractions for others who seek to learn it. Its popularity does not derive from innate qualities that make it easy to learn. Although the student of English escapes the complications of linguistic gender and prefix mutation common in many other languages, they still have to tackle the myriad variations of pronunciation and spelling, and acquire the potentially enormous vocabulary. While learning English may have economic and educational benefits, its popularity is largely derived from the fact that it is the nearest thing to a world language that exists. The other feature commonly cited as contributing to its increasing use, is its adaptability. Kachru has suggested that 'one reason for this dominance of English is its propensity for acquiring new identities, its power of assimilation, its adaptability to 'decolonization' as a language, its manifestation in a range of varieties, and above all its suitability as a flexible medium for literary and other types of creativity across languages and cultures (cited in Baugh and Cable, 1993). This is most readily seen in the phenomenal vocabulary of English and the ease with which neologisms (new words) are coined and loan words borrowed from other languages. However, the most significant aspect of the English language is not its popularity and adaptability, but the fact that it seems **normal** to those for whom it is their first and only language. This comfortable feeling with one's own language, is easily translated into an assumption of its naturalness; thus the ideological belief in its superiority is reinforced by the seemingly natural fact that so many other people from other countries also wish to use it.

The assumption of normality

Accompanying this perception of normality is a series of assumptions about English and other languages. For example, it is commonly assumed by English speakers that all words in one language have a matching word and concept in another. This is the assumption that all languages describe a universal reality, which all humans share. While this type of congruency can been mapped to some extent in the words used to describe the physical world, it is not the case for the social, emotional and intellectual realms of society and self. As noted in the previous chapter, the nomenclature of different family structures, of emotional states and of intellectual ideas shows considerable variation in how these things may be conceptualized and described. This notion of an objective external reality represented directly through language in our minds was challenged in the 18th century by the philosopher Hume (1740), was further undermined in the 19th by the psychologist James (1890) and has been comprehensively rejected in the 20th century by phenomenologists like Husserl (1970) and Schutz (1972). They contend the impossibility of experiencing the world other than subjectively, that is, through our own sensory perceptions of it. Consequently, rather than a single universal reality, there is a multiplicity of experience and subjective interpretation, resulting in multiple realities. As we shall see later in this chapter, the notion of a fixed common reality shared by all, in which it is believed that words in different languages are describing the same fundamental world, is inherently ethnocentric because it denies the possibility of cultural variation.

Probably the most significant assumption is that of the superiority of the English language. This may be viewed explicitly in terms of its utility but more saliently arises from the implicit assumption of the naturalness of English culture, values and attitudes for those who are raised within it. Those who grow up with the language rarely have occasion to examine carefully how their language carries ideas about the world and their place within it. As Steiner has noted, 'we are so much the product of set feeling patterns, Western culture has so thoroughly stylized our perceptions, that we experience our "traditionality" as natural. In particular we leave unquestioned the historical causes, the roots of determinism which underlie the "recursive" structure of our sensibility and expressive codes' (cited in Husband, 1977).

This assumption of traditionality leaves most people unaware of the social forces which have shaped their language. They simply take for granted the apparent normality that it carries within it and is represented by its use. It is this **naturalness** that Saussure's pioneering work undermined when he suggested that the concepts and categories that we use to describe our world are human creations rather than immutable representations of the real world.

Outside of formal linguistics some of the most challenging analyses of what language means and how it is used have been undertaken by people who have been marginalized in some way and thus have cause to examine the ways in which society operates to disadvantage them. Feminists who reject the use of generic masculine words like 'his' and 'mankind', and have sometimes created alternatives like 'herstory' to replace 'history', while making the point that the traditional use of English is one which renders women and their achievements invisible (Spender, 1980). The critical analysis of language is often focused upon contentious moral and political ideas. Opponents of nuclear arms have highlighted the euphemistic blandness of the language which masks the intentions of those who promote them. Terms like 'potential', 'neutralize' and 'target efficiency', actually refer to the death-making capacities of weapons intended to kill people but disguise and sanitize this crucial fact in the technocratic jargon of military management. Debates about other issues such as abortion and euthanasia are inevitably concerned with the meaning of words like 'choice', 'life' and 'freedom'. The proponents argue about what life is and when it begins and ends, who has choice and whose body it is that they are referring to.

Linguistic variation

Within Western traditions of thought, the concept of a dichotomy, of a distinction between two elements, is a common analytical device. One version of this device is the notion of knowledge as a dynamic progression from thesis to antithesis to synthesis. This idea dates from ancient Greece and from this, in the writings of Feurbach, Hegel and Marx, has developed a tradition of dialectical analysis. In folk wisdom, less sophisticated versions of the idea of duality are embodied in everyday language and have become some of the most dominant ways of thinking about the world and ordering our perceptions of it. For many people this seems a natural way of thinking about things: day and night, good and bad, true or false, black or white, land or sea, and so on. However, there is a crucial difference between the dialectical model and models of duality as ways of making sense of the world; this difference can have significant consequences for people who may be thus categorized. Whereas the dialectical model presupposes conflict between opposing ideas or elements, it ultimately enjoins the thinker to reconcile the opposing elements into some form of synthesis and so does not favour either of the two elements, since both are necessary elements of a dynamic progression. The duality model simply defines one element in terms of the other. For example, night is defined, most simply, as the absence of daylight.

The relevance of this apparently unrelated excursion is threefold. First, this is a model of making sense of the world that is essentially relational – that is, one category of person, animal or object is defined in relation to another; thus land is not water, an animal is not a mineral and so on. Definition is the act of distinction, recognition and categorization of some element of difference; in the preceding example, solidity, liquidity and animation could be the defining criteria. Definition might not be problematic if the categories and criteria that we used were directly derived from an objective real world, but if there is no such world then we have to accept that these categories are essentially social constructions. Thus, they are open to influence, change and reinterpretation. Cameron (1992) has persuasively analysed how such 'binary oppositions' have contributed to the discrimination of women, and observes that 'the urge to dichotomise is a product of indoctrination and not a native habit'. For example, the distinction between male and female may be made on the basis of chromosomal difference and genitalia, which is arguably an objective and scientific distinction. However, when making the distinction of gender between men and women, the criteria are obviously social creations, involving notions of femininity and masculinity, which are typically sets of idealized characteristics that each sex is supposed to possess, such as motherliness, tenderness, bravery, aggression, and so on.

The history of sexuality provides another example of how such dualities can be socially constructed: the distinction made between homosexual and heterosexual is not absolute and has not always been differentiated in the past. Even today the meaning varies, so that in some Mediterranean cultures, men who sexually penetrate other men do not perceive themselves as homosexual; that distinction is reserved for those men who prefer to be anally penetrated. Furthermore, the assumption that the dichotomous categories are invariably mutually exclusive may lead to a misreading or misunderstanding of the person or things referred to – by presenting a static view of them or by simply failing to recognize some other potential element of differentiation or significance. What seems real or natural is simply the set of definitions and categories that we learn through socialization and subsequently iterate and reiterate through our actions and thoughts. The question of how we may selectively alter and change these categories is considered in Chapter 7 in the discussion on power; for the moment it is sufficient to recognize the powerful consequences of duality models.

The second point is that such simplistic forms of definition tend by their very nature to exaggerate the differences between two elements when it might seem more logical in some circumstances to recognize similarities. How different are the Welsh from the English or the Scots? The main point is that the ways in which people distinguish their world through their language provides a crucial indication of how they see themselves and others. Sociologists such as Durkheim (1938) long ago recognized how such distinctions perform an important function in creating group identity, and explained how they may have negative consequences for those who are defined as different. This aspect of social differentiation and identity is discussed further in the following chapter.

The third point is that such binomial distinctions frequently carry evaluative judgements within them, that is judgements of preference and worth. Thus the duality becomes skewed with one element being the dominant signifier or marker of definition. This is particularly noticeable in the way in which monoglot English speakers typically view other languages or variations from their own dialect, accent or form of English. Once the assumption of normality has been made, it is common for variations away from the assumed norm to be seen not simply as different but as abnormal and inferior. Thus the norm is not a statistical average but an ideological one, since it presents one feature as the baseline from which other features are then differentiated. This approach leads to the devaluation of that which is different, and to thus potentially to the pathologization of those who possess supposedly 'abnormal' characteristics. For example, despite the evidence which shows that homosexuality has been a feature of human sexuality since accounts of social life were first recorded, heterosexuality is often presented as being the sexual norm; thus homosexuality, instead of being seen simply as one form of sexuality, is derogated. It is only comparatively recently that it has been removed from categorization as a form of mental illness and there are still people living in institutions whose original grounds for admission was their supposedly 'abnormal' homosexuality.

Frequently, alterations in work practices or policies that seek to promote equal opportunities are undermined by contrasting the proposed changes against an assumed conception of normality; so that the changes are viewed as an aberration or threat to normal affairs. The phrase 'promoting Welsh' may be used to describe a Welsh language initiative as if English were the norm for all people, whereas for approximately 20% of the population of Wales it is not. In contrast, the fact that most Welsh speakers are faced daily with situations where English is assumed to be the norm is rarely described as 'promoting English'. In practice, as Williams (1994) has noted, even when language becomes an issue, English is often used as the sole linguistic qualification even when this is not appropriate. He describes the uncritical use of this criterion in a report on the recruitment of French social workers in the London Borough of Newham, where it was stated that the interviewing panel was impressed by one prospective employee, but advised her to 'brush up on her English'. No apparent consideration was made of the numerous other languages spoken in the Borough; as Williams comments, 'The English requirement is normal, unmarked'. Fishman (1988) has noted a similar presumption with regard to the use of English within the USA. As we shall see in Chapter 5, such implicit assumptions, which favour one group at the expense of others, can be maintained by a cultural hegemony, which obscures or 'normalizes' unfair practices.

Even variation within the English language may be seen as abnormal, so that differences of accent, dialect and grammar are viewed negatively as being inferior to an assumed standard of written and spoken English. In their efforts to determine the National Curriculum and set educational standards for English in schools, the Conservative Governments of the 1980s and 1990s echoed many of the mistaken premises of earlier efforts to define proficiency in English. Both the Newbolt Report (1921) and the Spens Report (1938) perceived regional dialects and common patterns of vernacular speech as being indicative of slovenliness, poor education and inadequacy. The work of Bernstein (1973), who posited that working-class children operated with a more restricted form of language than their middle-class counterparts and consequently did less well at school, has also been misrepresented as evidence of the need to ensure that all children should be taught standard English and should strive to emulate Received Pronunciation.

These assumptions of inferiority are, however, not supported by sociolinguistic research; the work undertaken by Tizard and Hughes (1984) and Wells (1987) does not support this view. Similar assumptions of inferiority have also been expressed in the USA and the UK about the language used by young black people, where the use of slang, Creole and patois is perceived as an inferior linguistic form indicative of a general lack of language skills. At one time in the USA it was speculated that black people were incapable of speaking 'proper' English because of the supposed limits of their physiognomy and restricted intelligence (Trudgill, 1984)! Such views represent a failure to appreciate that, apart from the common variations arising from social class and geography, the deliberate switching of language can be a dissociative measure used by social groups who feel marginalized and devalued (Giles et al., 1977; Pugh, 1994b). This aspect of language use is pursued further in the next chapter.

There is a long history of sexist and negative stereotypes of women and language; it has been variously stated that women's voices are harsh and strident, or soft and polite, that their spoken English is incomplete and patchy, and that their use of language reflects a general inability to think in abstract terms; in short, that they are less logical than men and are thus inferior. But, as Cameron (1992) points out, even the differences in speech styles revealed by research may not be indicative of innate difference but instead reflect the social position of women in patriarchal societies – where women have fewer opportunities to use and rehearse formal speech styles, where they may be able to leave more things unsaid in conversation because they may 'assume a great deal of shared knowledge and cooperation'. They may be more egalitarian in their conversational 'rules', and take turns and interrupt each other less in conversation, because of their recognition of shared social position and lack of personal confidence. The question of shared speech context is developed further in Chapter 4.

Much of the evidence on turn-taking and interruption in conversation which appears to show patterns of male dominance and female submissiveness is based upon small unrepresentative samples from a limited range of social situations and should be treated cautiously (Ellis and Beattie, 1986). While these results may fit with our presumptions, it is difficult to judge how accurate these observations are as indicators of general speech patterns. What is well established is that in many languages there is a tendency for women to use higher status forms of pronunciation than men in situations where careful speech is required. It has been suggested that this derives from greater linguistic sensitivity, that is, that women are used to having to fit in with more dominant patterns in most things in their lives and language is simply another one of these. Alternatively, working-class women may have more opportunity to acquire and rehearse these higher prestige variants because of the broader social contact gained in their types of service employment in shops and offices, whereas working-class men are more likely to work with other men of the same background.

The prevailing view within sociolinguistics is that there is no basis for assuming any reduced capacity in the ability of different languages and dialects to perform all of the necessary communicative functions within the social group. The idea that some dialects or languages are linguistically superior to others is simply not a tenable proposition (Crystal, 1987). Looking further afield, the related notion that so called 'primitive people' spoke primitive languages has also been shown to be mistaken. Sapir (1921) demonstrated that the assumption that they spoke only in concrete terms and lacked a clear grammar and structure to their languages was erroneous. Therefore we should make a clear distinction between the social and political ideas about language and the accompanying beliefs that such variations reflect the intrinsic worth of different languages and their actual linguistic and communicative properties. As Crystal (1987) states:

> Some languages are of course more useful or prestigious than others, at a given period of history, but this is due to the pre-eminence of the speakers at that time, and not due to any inherent linguistic characteristics. The view of modern linguistics is that a language should not be valued on the basis of the political or economic influence of its speakers.
>
> *Crystal, 1987*

This quotation nicely establishes the point that ideas about language are primarily social judgements rather than technical facts. This is a critical point because it locates the debate about the status of languages firmly in the social and political sphere and removes the question of technical merit. However, Crystal's statement does not adequately establish the basis for the 'prestige', which is more accurately described as being a consequence of power rather than 'pre-eminence'. The relationship of power to language is explored further in Chapter 5.

Thinking of variations from or within English as abnormal or inferior forms ignores the historical and sociolinguistic reality of language use. Britain has never been an entirely monolingual society with a pure and standardized language. Until Samuel Johnson's first dictionary in 1755 there was no common agreement as to how to spell many words, let alone pronounce them. Regional accents and dialects remained common for all social classes, only finally being replaced in the upper and middle classes by standard English and Received Pronunciation in the early years of this century. Even today it is been estimated that less than 10% of the population speaks standard English and that even fewer speak it with the Received Pronunciation characteristically associated with BBC broadcasters (Hughes and Trudgill, 1978). As Ellis and Beattie (1986) have noted, contemporary English displays remarkable changes from the forms in classical texts such as Beowulf (10th century) and those used by Shakespeare (16th century).

Besides the existing older languages of Gaelic, Irish and Welsh, there is a surprising diversity of languages spoken in Britain. The Language Census of London schools (ILEA, 1987) discovered that there were 172 different languages spoken by children in the capital. Other broader surveys of language diversity, such as the Linguistic Minorities Project (1985) and the work of Alladina and Edwards (1991) have also established the extent and diversity of non-English languages; it is evident that the assumption that Britain is a mono-lingual state is inaccurate.

Monolingualism, nation and culture

Despite the fact that multilingualism is more common throughout the world than monolingualism, the notion that one nation equals one language is still widespread. This idea came to prominence with the 19th-century enthusiasm for nationalism, with its emphasis upon common heritage. The political signifi-cance of the rise of nationalism has been extensively documented, Anderson (1983), for example, describes most of the efforts towards nationalism as attempts to 'achieve solidarities on an essentially imagined basis'. The construc-tion of ideologies of nationalism that rely heavily upon language to define the group are still prevalent in this century. When the new state of Israel was formed the dead language of Hebrew was resurrected to establish and mark the new nation. New nation-states frequently attempt to standardize one dominant language, ostensibly for reasons of efficiency in communication, government and education, but primarily, they can be viewed either as attempts to create a uniform identity, a sense of commonality and belonging, or as attempts by one linguistic group to establish its predominance over another.

The widespread assumption in Britain that eventually the older languages like Welsh and Gaelic would disappear was matched by a similar view, held throughout the post-war years, that all incomers would lose their own language as they 'naturally' learnt English. This was based not solely upon the pragmatic necessity of them doing so, but upon an assumption of the superiority of the English language and hence, of the desirability of them doing so. The assimilationist model of race relations assumes that immigrants could and should 'fit in', by learning English and abandoning their original languages and culture (Cashmore and Troyna, 1983). When Margaret Thatcher spoke of fears of 'swamping' it was widely interpreted that she was cynically playing the 'race card'. This stratagem is not simply a reference to the number of immigrants or their colour, but also refers to some notion of cultural purity and social homogeneity. This notion requires further examination because it illustrates the highly static concept of culture embedded within this type of thinking.

From the earliest times the impact of trade, war and colonization have led either to the replacement of one language by another or the shaping of older languages by those of the incomers (Baugh and Cable, 1993). For example, Welsh could lay a stronger claim than English to be the 'proper' language of the British Isles since it derives from the older Brythonic tongue. The impact of colonization can be seen, for example, in Roman place-names such as Blandford Forum (market), Upton Magna (greater), and in the legacy of loan words within the Welsh language, such as 'pont' (bridge), 'eglwys' (church). As even a cursory glance at an etymological dictionary of English will show, words such as 'algebra', 'assassin', 'bungalow', 'dandelion', 'curry' and 'paper' merely represent the tip of the iceberg of external influence upon English language and culture. English not only originates from an Indo-European family of languages which includes Sanskrit, but has been successively altered by Latin, by various Scandinavian languages and by Norman French (Baugh and Cable, 1993). The notion that countries have 'pure' cultures represented by the unchanging homogeneity of their language and population is for most countries a myth – a mistaken, ahistorical and unsociological assumption (Jenks, 1993). Nevertheless, this myth is powerful, and debates and struggles over what children should be taught in school often reflect this mistaken conception. As Said (1993) has noted: 'defensive, reactive, and even paranoid nationalism is, alas, frequently woven into the very fabric of education, where children as well as older students are taught to venerate and celebrate the uniqueness of **their** tradition (usually and invidiously at the expense of others)'.

The myth of national monoculture is often reiterated to provide comfort and assurance in the face of social change. It may be used to deny the just claims and rights of linguistic and cultural minorities. It is no accident that the success of Fascism in Europe during the 1920s and 1930s was partly based upon romanticized myths – myths which in the German version, Nazism, referred to the disaggregation and former greatness of the Aryan peoples and their supposed common inheritance and culture. Incorporating the erroneous belief that culture was genetically transmitted, the Fascists found confirmation of their ideas in the work of Gobineau, who believed that some 'races' were stronger and more successful than others because of the purity of their blood; consequently, intermarriage between 'races' was held to be the cause of the weakness of the inferior 'races' (Kedward, 1969; Mosse, 1966).

Such mistaken views ignore the fact that all the major European languages bear the marks of other cultures, and minimizes the extent to which most cultures are an amalgam of historical influences. Defence of the mythical purity of language is often a rallying point for social conservatives because, as Cameron (1992) succinctly states, it 'is related to the way in which people think of language as a fixed point in the flux of experience and cling to the certainties they feel are embodied in language'. However, a review of the history of such diverse aspects of social life as technology, farming, music, politics, religion, clothing and food, reveals a succession of changes and innovations. In the last 30 years, the acceptance in Britain of food dishes from other cultures, such as spaghetti, hamburgers, curry, pizza and chow mein, indicates the rapid pace of cultural change. Pearson (1983) describes the remarkable similarity in the language used, over the years, to condemn the perceived excesses of youth. He notes the rhetoric which bemoans the speech, dress and behaviour of young people, and reveals the older generation's yearning for a mythical past, an era of peace, stability and contentment. Changes in culture can be perceived in virtually every area of social life. For example, within nursing and medicine the influence of different cultural ideas of health has become more widespread with the realization that holistic conceptions may offer more comprehensive models of health and dysfunction. Likewise, there is a growing acceptance of the fact that some alternative therapies may bring positive benefits, such as the use of acupuncture for pain relief, meditation and yoga for relaxation and stress reduction. The growing acceptance is signalled by the renaming of these therapeutic alternatives as 'complementary' medicine, though the phrase itself still confirms the predominance of the medical perspective.

Returning to the central issue of attitudes to languages, it is important to recognize that there are very few countries in the world which are purely monolingual; virtually all states have significant minorities who speak older indigenous tongues or have migrants who have brought their own languages with them. Failure to acknowledge this diversity denies the multilingual reality which pertains in most societies and hence, as we shall see later, tends to devalue people who use the 'non-standard' minority languages.

Bilingualism

The Rampton (1981) and Cox Reports (Department of Education and Science and Welsh Office, 1988) looked at the issue of children learning English as a second language; both reports exhorted teachers to avoid devaluing the child's first language and instead use it to support learning. Despite these recommendations, contemporary thinking about bilingualism is confused and continues to undermine the first language of non-English speakers. Commenting upon the Swann Report (1985), Pattanayak (1991) noted that it 'rejected the twin ideas of bilingual education and mother tongue maintenance as a single educational aim. This ambivalence has resulted in favouring a selective elite bilingualism, while resisting bilingualism for minority language speakers'. The present situation is one in which certain languages (mostly European), such as English, French and German, are perceived to be more useful or valuable than others. Consequently the languages of many of Britain's minority groups, such as Urdu, Panjabi, Hindi and Vietnamese, have less status and are regarded as inferior and less useful. It may be that these judgements rest primarily upon an estimation of the economic value of the respective languages but underpinning these judgements are ethnocentric assumptions about culture and the value of bilingualism *per se*. Fishman (1988) notes that the use of the term 'bilingual' in the USA is almost unique in its pejorative connotation of 'non-English mother tongue', by which he means the implication that the bilingual is a low-status immigrant. Fishman argues that the Anglification of millions of immigrants and native Americans has been accomplished without any formal statement to the effect that English should be the national language. Even the Bilingual Education Act 1968 did not seek to preserve existing minority languages, but presumed the desirability and predominance of English; the implicit intention being to improve a child's English to the point where it could be the language for education. This, however, may disadvantage children whose first language is not English. A study in Florida of a programme to assist Spanish-speaking schoolchildren learn English (Rivero and Brice, 1994) examined the assumption that there was a strong interdependence between academic proficiency displayed through one language and performance displayed through a second learned language; they found that while there was a link, it was a weak one. However, in other countries, the status of 'bilingual' is not only regarded as 'normal', but may be positively valued: the growing popularity of Welsh-medium schools in Wales is but one example of this.

The belief that at a social level language is 'a zero-sum game (if I have more of it, you have less)' (Cameron, 1992) is essentially a belief that language is a fixed commodity which it is necessary to compete for, and that it is ultimately susceptible to control. This reification of language as a resource is also seen at the personal level where the capacity of children to learn language is frequently assumed to be fixed (Bellin, 1994). Baker (1992) has pointed out that, when considering this issue, many monoglot English speakers assume that a situation of competition exists, where one language is presumed to be a threat to the other: 'Positive consequences for one language imply negative consequences for the other language. This gives the impression of languages existing in a kind of balance.' Superficially, this view appears to be borne out by language testing of bilingual people, which shows that few have equal competence in all areas of both languages, such as formal and informal speech, writing, vocabulary and grammar. Baker suggests that this leads to a negative 'deficiency model' of bilingualism, in which it is believed that two languages cannot mutually exist together in the same person or society. Thus children learning one language, for example, do so at the expense of another. This view presumes a limited capacity for learning language, or assumes that at a wider social level the use of a minority language is to the detriment of the majority language. He cites Grosjean (1985) who stresses 'how negative – often destructive – the monolingual view of bilingualism has been, and in many areas still is'.

Following Grosjean (1989) Baker argues that the 'measurement of a bilingual's competence can only be achieved by examining the total language repertoire enacted in varying domains'. He contends that the supposed deficits are not in fact negative features, but reflections of the fact that, where people regularly use two languages, they typically use them in different settings (**domains**) according to the requirements of the situation. The way a bilingual individual learns and adapts language to different situations is thus highly specific to that person's experience. Though there are some typical patterns of usage within the UK and the USA, the non-English first language is typically used as the language of the home and of informal social life, while English is reserved for more formal situations, such as work and education (Alladina and Edwards, 1991). Thus, the tested competence of bilingual speakers simply reflects the skill levels necessary to function effectively in different domains. Baker's contention that the most effective learning is that which is required to function in any given situation echoes Illich's (1973) view of learning and knowledge. Failure to grasp the 'situated' or contextual nature of language skills often results in negative attitudes towards bilingualism, as the bilingual person is often assessed from a monolingual frame of comparison instead of a bilingual one: 'The bilingual is not two monolinguals in one frame, but a unity uniquely different from a monolingual...to be bicultural is not to own two monocultures. The way two cultures are blended, harmonized and combined is unique and not simply the sum of two parts' (Baker, 1992).

Therefore, the assumption of equal competence in both languages is usually inaccurate because it fails to recognize how language use is structured by the demands of different domains, and similarly the assumption that lack of competence in one language is representative of overall linguistic competence is also misleading. Gumperz (1982a, b) has confirmed how monolinguals from the dominant language groups in societies construe difficulties in communication with linguistic minorities as evidence of the social and intellectual inadequacy of the minority language speakers. This attitude can also be seen when English monoglot speakers hear what they perceive to be English words within the bilingual person's non-English first-language and assume that these words reveal a linguistic deficit. This perception fails to recognize that most languages adopt loan words from other languages, and overlooks the possibility that the words may in fact originate from the bilingual person's first language, or possibly derive from a third language common to both, such as French or Latin.

Attitudes towards bilingualism are often most apparent when issues of employment and qualification arise with regard to people whose first language is not English. Attitudes towards Asian doctors and nurses may reveal racist and ethnocentric linguistic ideas that have little basis in fact. The question of effective communication is certainly one that should be addressed for all people within the helping services, but it is frequently only raised for some prospective employees, and often without clear criteria of competence. Assuming that all English first-language speakers are competent and that all non-English first-language bilinguals are not is clearly a discriminatory attitude and may serve to disguise or 'make respectable' other more fundamental stereotypical prejudices against those who are culturally different from the dominant grouping. As Davies (1994) has noted, we should remember that 'bilingualism contains a wide variety of control over language; [that] very few people have a balanced control and equal abilities in two languages; [and that] bilingual people tend to feel more comfortable in one language than the other'.

Whether they feel confident or not will depend upon their ability within a given language, their power relative to other persons within a particular situation, the status of their first language and the existence of any conventions or 'rules' within the situation. It is clear that, if minority speakers wish to use their preferred language, the question of choice is not a simple one. These issues are discussed further in Chapters 5 and 7.

Finally, it should be noted that, when migration or other social changes necessitate learning a second language, men may have severe reservations about women learning the new language. The experience of some immigrants into Britain has shown how threatening this can be to male perceptions of appropriate gender roles. The significant factors appear to be the extent to which men and women are able to replicate their traditional roles in the new society with regard to employment and home life. Zentella (1987) has noted how women in the Puerto Rican community in New York experience a conflict of roles, being expected to mediate with the English-speaking world and yet to act to maintain traditional culture within the family. Former US colleagues of mine have remarked upon the skill with which these conflicts are handled by younger, unmarried women, who adapt their dress, speech and behaviour quite consciously according to the situations they are in.

ATTITUDES IN LANGUAGE

Taboo words and ideas

Distinct from the attitudes held **about** particular languages are the attitudes expressed **in** language. These are expressed through the ascriptive value attached to words used, that is, whether they are approving or disapproving of someone or something, and by the way in which they are used or expressed. As noted earlier in this chapter, actual changes in the literal and symbolic meanings attached to words will also reflect important shifts in attitudes and behaviour within a society. This is most obvious when we examine the different **taboo words** used by different people and different societies. Taboo words refer to ideas or behaviours that are socially prohibited or restricted in some way and are thus not for general or everyday use. In the English language the most common taboo words relate to sex and bodily functions such as intercourse, menstruation and excretion. It is generally supposed by many linguists and anthropologists that taboo words are indicative of some of the things most feared or prized by particular societies but, as Cameron (1992) notes, the taboo words about women and their bodies may be more accurately explained as an indication of derogatory male attitudes regarding women's inferiority. This is also reflected in the greater taboo strength in English attached to 'female' swear words: to be called a 'prick' may be insulting but is not generally regarded as offensive as the female equivalent, 'cunt'. Of course, ambivalent male attitudes to women's sexuality are also apparent in the use of words like 'slag', which have no similarly derogatory male equivalent. There may be variations in taboo strength even within similar cultures. In France, for example, the phrase '*petit con*', literally 'little cunt', is widely used in everyday speech, even by children.

Nevertheless, whatever the underlying explanation for the taboo value attached to particular words, their use is normally hedged with intricate social rules. Typically, they may only be referred to obliquely, or used by particular people in particular situations. The use of taboo words in the wrong setting or by the wrong person is often thought to bring bad luck or be indicative of disregard of social conventions and the feelings of others. Trudgill (1983) notes how bilingual speakers will avoid using words from their second language which sound like taboo words from their mother tongue. He reports that this process can work in both directions, with speakers also avoiding words from their first language which sound similar to taboo words in English.

Another type of taboo common in many societies is the use of secret names and diminutives. These stem from beliefs that others can bring bad luck or control a person by the knowledge of their name; thus a secret or private name is used as a protective device and is known only by the closest relatives or friends. One version of this type of taboo is related by Mary Crow Dog (1991), who tells how on the birth of her first child she should have sought a *winkte*, a male homosexual, to give her baby a secret name. The Lakota Sioux believed that gay men lived a long time and that the secret names they conferred would also confer longevity upon the child. The power of naming is still evident: for many Muslims the offence given by Salman Rushdie originates from the taking of their God's name in vain. Even in so called advanced, Westernized societies, as Crystal (1987) has suggested, few would consider it appropriate to name a new ship the *Titanic*!

Most societies have found ways of dealing with taboo words and ideas by the use of euphemisms and avoidance (Ayto, 1993). Instead of referring to a woman's vagina and womb, I heard one doctor use the phrase 'down there', and many patients still refer to their rectum and anus as their 'back passage'. Avoidance of taboo behaviour such as incest is maintained in some societies by men either avoiding contact with female relatives or by the use of ritualized forms of speech which remind both parties of the particular restrictions in their relationship towards each other. See Chapter 4, especially the reference to Henslin and Briggs's (1971) study of the rituals of gynaecological examinations.

Until relatively recently within health services it was often taboo to mention death directly to patients; ostensibly this was done to protect the patient from the awful realization of their own demise, but arguably it was the medical professionals who were being protected too, since proof of the limitations and imminent failure of their own knowledge and skills was looming. Furthermore, to engage directly with another in the confronting and acceptance of the likelihood of their death was emotionally challenging and threatened the protective distance that normally shields professionals from the pain and conflict inherent in their job (Satyamurti, 1979). This detachment, of course, is often deliberately sought and perceived as being a valued characteristic of 'professional' practice. The consequences of this distancing have been criticized by the founders of the hospice movement, who have shown how the taboo on discussing death leads to a neglect of important issues of pain relief and control and of the necessity of preparation for death, and thus obstructs the provision of the care and support that can be given when the resources of technology and curative medicine have proved ineffective.

In the field of child protection the presence of social taboos on discussing sexual behaviour and the sexual parts of the body may also lead to inadequate services. Workers who are unprepared to hear the reality of sexual abuse of children, or are uncomfortable with the use of taboo words, may through their shocked responses communicate their own discomfort to the child who is disclosing abuse to them. The worker's personal distaste and disgust may be interpreted by the victim as pertaining to them personally rather than to the behaviour of the perpetrator, and so may inhibit the helping processes of sharing and ventilation, as well as obstructing the collection of information vital to the task of protection.

Similarly, the professional helper who is unprepared for and unfamiliar with the use of euphemisms for subjects may miss the significance of what is being conveyed to them. For example, a child's statement that 'I don't like my uncle, he's got a worm that comes into my bed at night', might indicate rather more than a vivid imagination. Insensitivity to the power of taboo may also lead to a worker using language that shocks or offends the client.

Changing attitudes

While the power of taboo words is frequently invoked in swearing, when words like 'fuck' and 'cunt' are used to indicate strength of feeling or power, in some circumstances even these have lost much of their power to shock, though as with all such words the context and the form of expression remain the important variables. The more frequent public use of such words is one linguistic indicator of social change. It is clear from the initial outrage that greeted the first recorded use of the word 'fuck' in British broadcasting that attitudes towards English slang words for sexual intercourse have become more liberal, though this also varies from one language to another.

Changing attitudes are most noticeable when examining the terminology used to describe hitherto marginalized, different or disadvantaged groups. When homosexuals in the USA began using the word 'gay' they were attempting to create a new more positive identity for themselves. Latterly, some gay men and women have taken the word 'queer' and are seeking to redefine it positively. The sixties slogan 'Say it loud, I'm black and I'm proud' is another example of a conscious attempt to move away from the use of the word 'negro' and confront the essential fact of differentiation, in this case skin colour. Such has been the success of this changing nomenclature, that for white people to use the term 'negro' is regarded as insulting, not polite. This strategy of reclaiming and recreating language has become extensively used by other disadvantaged groups who have sought to redefine their position within society (Pugh, 1994b).

For example, the People First movement is not simply aiming to replace the terms 'mental handicap' and 'retardation' with the phrases 'people with learning difficulties/learning disabilities', but is attempting to redefine the conceptual model used to understand mental impairment and its social consequences. The movement explicitly rejects a medical model based upon the concept of deficiency, and instead focuses upon the practical problems of learning and analytically views the concept of disability as a social label or consequence of the social response to the initial impairment. Hence the problems of people with learning difficulties are redefined not as problems of genetic damage or brain trauma, but as problems caused by the social response to the people who have such impairments. The real problems of poor institutional care, poverty and stigmatization derive not from the physical causes of their impairments but from our society's behaviour towards such people. Conflicts about meaning and values are discussed further in Chapter 5; for the moment it is sufficient to recognize that explicit attempts to change words are attempts to change meanings and ideas, and so may be viewed as struggles over power – the power to define and to label.

The most telling examination of how words and language reflect attitudes and shape them has come from the feminist analyses of the interaction of gender and language (Spender, 1980; Cameron, 1990, 1992; Coates, 1993). While the salient ideas about power will be discussed further in Chapter 5, the genesis of contemporary feminist interest in language, as noted earlier in this chapter, originates in the critique of the representation of women within Western cultures, and with concern about sexist forms of language, which represent a masculine world as normal and generic, and largely ignore or misrepresent women. This critique is predominantly concerned with the ways in which men's and women's views of themselves and each other are conditioned by language and the images conveyed by it (Cameron, 1992). The strongest form of such linguistic determinism lies in the work of Spender (1980), who contends that women are alienated by having to use a language that has been constructed by men and that in language, as in many other aspects of society, women are disadvantaged.

Coates (1993) develops a different theme within her work, mainly focusing upon the history of ideas of difference between men's and women's language, and she provides a broad review of contemporary evidence of differentiation in language use and speech behaviour. Coates's conclusion is that there are significant differences, in that language 'reflects and reinforces' existing categories of gender and that these differences are replicated through education and other forms of social behaviour, to the continuing disadvantage of women.

Cameron (1990, 1992) attempts to develop a distinctive feminist analysis and critique of linguistic theories from the sometimes difficult position of an academic linguist and committed feminist. Her work is distinguished by a very clear exposition of existing theories and a candid account of the development of her ideas. Cameron is especially interested in situating theories of language within a model of society which adequately captures the extent to which the human actor is both determined and determining, that is, is created by her/his experiences and in turn having the agency to act upon the world – a theme which was introduced in Chapter 1 of this book and is developed further in Chapter 5. All three writers, however, concur in the main with the conclusion – that language reflects and constructs existing forms of gender dominance and disadvantage.

CONCLUSION

For the purpose of clarity this chapter has made a distinction between attitudes to language and attitudes in language. This helps to distinguish between attitudes about particular languages and by inference the people who use them, and attitudes expressed in and through language, that is, implied or conveyed by the actual words used about a subject. Of course, in general speech both may be conveyed together and given added force by forms of variation such as intonation and emphasis. This review of how attitudes and language relate to each other indicates the importance of thinking of language in a broader context than most linguists have hitherto done. Issues of power and identity cannot be satisfactorily discussed without reference to questions such as who uses particular languages, what factors influence their choice of language, who holds power, who benefits and who does not. These issues are developed in the following chapters; at this stage the crucial point of relevance to the development of practice is to recognize that many of us may have a considerable degree of rethinking to do about our assumptions about language. A conscious awareness of where we are coming from, in terms of our own attitudes about language, is a critical foundation for an informed professional practice that seeks to challenge discrimination. It is the first step in the process which Dominelli (1988) calls **conscientization**, a 'process whereby individuals make connections between the social relations they endorse and perpetuate through their attitudes, values and behaviour and the social positions they occupy'.

Language and identity

3

For you are never so smart again in a language learned in middle age nor
so romantic or brave or kind. All the best of you is in the old tongue, but
when you speak your best in America you become a yokel, a dumb
Norskie, and when you speak English, an idiot.

Keillor, 1985

Yan said, Doctors are assholes these days. It's all about power. Everyone
wants to show off their power.

Min, 1993

INTRODUCTION

The first quotation could stand for the experience of millions of adult migrants,
who have felt that the best of themselves was in the old tongue, their identity
inescapably bound up with their first language and their second remaining a
continuous reminder of not quite fitting in, of not being themselves, because
their sense of their true self is not reflected in their imprecise grasp of the new
tongue (Baker, Arseneault and Gallant, 1994). This sense of displacement
together with the feeling of being caught between two cultures is a common
theme throughout autobiographical accounts and fictional renditions of the
experience of transition and second language acquisition. Clearly, the degree of
competence in a new language has a direct bearing on the sense of ease experienced within a new country, but there is a deeper process than this. The second
quotation is from the autobiography of Anchee Min, who left China in 1984.
This book was written in her second language, English, which she felt gave her
the freedom to express feelings that she found difficult in her first language.
These feelings are bound up with the central issue of language and thought. As

the review in Chapter 1 concluded, whatever the level of determinism one attaches to language, there is little disagreement that it is a major factor in processing thought. Different languages reflect or construct different realities for people, and so logically it follows that language is a crucial mediator of identity. To assume that language is simply a means of communication is to ignore the relative nature of the world-view within different languages and to misunderstand the significance that it has for people as part of their self-image. However, the role of language in identity goes further than this, for as well as the differential world-views embodied within different languages and the self-conscious awareness of oneself as a speaker of this or that language, language mediates between the inner world of the person and the external world of other people. Language is the bridge that links us to the social world, but more than that, it constructs identity through its use; in one sense we find out and create who we are through the speaking of language.

LANGUAGE AS ONE FORM OF DIFFERENTIATION

Language is frequently ignored in discussions about equal opportunities or, if it is considered, it is tacked on as an afterthought together with other forms of difference such as religion and age. Language is rarely considered as an element of differentiation in its own right; more often it is simply subsumed as an aspect of 'race'. This conflation is highly problematic in terms of its consequences for people who use minority languages and rests upon some confused thinking about the idea of 'race'. What is usually signalled by the term is skin colour and hence language is perceived as an issue only when it refers to non-white people who do not speak English as their first language. However, the extensive range of language variation in terms of types and dialects undermines the simplistic assumption that language is simply a marginal aspect of 'race'. This absurd assumption ignores sign languages, the older tongues like Welsh and Gaelic, and the fact that there are large numbers of migrants and visitors to Britain whose first language is not English. Furthermore, the conflation of race and language has the effect of obscuring important differences between people who may appear to be the same but whose tribal group, religious caste or social class is additionally defined by their language. It should be remembered that bilingualism and multilingualism are the norm in many countries and the assumption that most countries are monocultural and monolingual is mistaken.

While the biological concept of 'race' is scientifically unsustainable, the term still has social meaning, in the sense that many people still believe and act as if there were separate 'races' (Mason, 1995; Rex, 1986). Miles (1989, 1993) argues that, because 'race' is an ideological construct which oppresses people, we should not use it, in order to avoid reinforcing or legitimizing it. An alternative way of referring to differences of colour, culture and language is to use the concept of ethnicity.

Ethnicity has been defined as 'all of the characteristics which go to make up cultural identity; origins, physical appearance, language, family structure, religious beliefs, politics, food, art, music, literature, attitudes towards the body, gender roles, clothing, education' (Storkey, 1991). This is similar to the definition of culture in Chapter 1. It differs most obviously in encompassing physical appearance among the list of characteristics, but this definition is deficient because it does not adequately reflect the self-conscious aspect of ethnicity. Ethnicity is about consciously shared self and group identity, the sense of group identity that derives from real or imagined similarities, which a group believes that it shares. In this sense, we are all ethnic, in that we are born, raised and live within a specific set of circumstances and in a culture that is not universal but is located in particular social classes, forms of education, patterns of religious belief, geographical places and so on (Thompson, 1993). This concept has the advantage of not reinforcing the mistaken notion of biologically distinct 'races' and encourages recognition of a multiplicity of forms of differentiation. It also avoids the tendency to minimize important differences between people: thus not all black people or women are the same, even if racists and misogynists think they are.

Ethnicity is thus often used as a way of avoiding the discredited term 'race', but many writers acknowledge the **social** significance of the idea and use the terms 'race' and 'ethnicity' interchangeably (Davis and Proctor, 1989). This, in my view, is a mistake because it tends to subsume all of the potential factors of differentiation and identity under one heading, usually skin colour. Nevertheless, using the concept of ethnicity uncritically is not without problems. As Mama (1992) has argued, ethnicity by 'focusing on the language, food, habits and clothing of black (African, Asian or Caribbean) people, masks and denies the fact of discrimination. Systematic and institutionalized racism is thereby reduced to cultural misunderstanding and is so depoliticized'. The simplistic substitution of the term 'ethnicity' for 'race' leads to what Mama terms the 'ethnicization' of the reality of discrimination based upon skin colour. The difficulty here is that even the concepts used to describe and analyse situations have a political significance, because they can focus attention in ways which may or may not highlight the problems facing particular groups. Just as the emphasis on 'race' can obscure important issues about language, so the concept of ethnicity can lead to a smokescreen of triviality, which obscures the central facts of racism and racial disadvantage arising from skin colour (Rex, 1986).

Nevertheless, as a means of understanding the complex and variable role of language in identity, the concept of ethnicity is valuable. What should be avoided is the simplistic conflation of 'race' with it – they are complementary terms of a different order. Whereas 'race' has no scientific validity, it does have considerable social meaning for people. Ethnicity, in contrast, is not widely used in general speech and, though it appears a more neutral term, its use too may have political implications. There is no need to champion the particular disadvantages that each term best illustrates, as if each were in competition for our attention; unfair practice is poor practice whomever it affects. Resources may be sought or policies pursued for one group at the expense of others, but the development of an analytical understanding of the multiplicity of disadvantage in our society does not necessitate a preemptive either/or choice. Each concept is a heuristic device, a way of thinking about things that is more or less useful according to our needs; like all social creations they can be selected, changed or dropped but neither should be treated as if it were exclusive, otherwise, as Thompson (1993) comments 'there is a danger in placing too much emphasis on the disparate elements of oppression and thus failing to see the links between, for example, racism and sexism, sexism and ageism and so on'.

While the concept of race is often used in a way that signals the belief that people are biologically different, the discrimination that accompanies it is often justified by reference to cultural and ethnic differences as much as the imagined physical ones. As Thompson aptly summarizes, 'race... is a social and political process whereby ethnic differences are translated into pseudo-biological racial deficits'.

Many of the assumptions about differences between people are not overt and explicit. Fishman (1977) has provided a useful analysis of what he called the 'unmobilized ethnicity' which underpins many ideas about bilingualism, some of which were described in Chapter 2. Other unmobilized assumptions can be seen in the misuse of the term 'ethnicity', which reveals the implicit conceptions of normality that some white people hold about themselves. For example, they may refer to older black people as 'ethnic elders', thus revealing their unspoken idea of what is the norm and what is an aberration from it, 'ethnic' in this context becoming a euphemism for 'black'. A more accurate use of the term might be 'ethnic minority elders' or 'black elders', because these directly convey the fact of difference from the white speaker instead of assuming a white baseline. This type of normative comparison, described in the previous chapter, is often used by people who do not intend to be racist or discriminatory but have not realized the extent to which their ethnocentric frame of reference reflects their particular social world. Without this understanding, perceptions of difference quickly become assumptions of deficit.

Ethnicity is not static: it may change from actions originating from within a group or from the group's response to external pressures. The two examples discussed later in this chapter indicate how language may be used to bind or define a group that feels under pressure. The relationship of language to ethnicity is a complex and variable one – it may be the core element which defines a group, as Edwards (1977) has noted: 'Language is important; it is a continuing bond and a potential rallying point for ethnic identity if required. However, in the absence of external pressures and in instances in which practical value is perceived to attach to identification with a larger society, language in its most communicative form is expendable.' Minority groups may persist and flourish even while the significance of their language diminishes if they do not perceive themselves as being under pressure. Karttunen (1977) in the USA has described how Finnish immigrants who experienced relatively few difficulties in adapting and being accepted in their new country quickly stopped using their native language because it served few useful functions for them.

WHAT IS IDENTITY?

The concept of identity has attracted much attention from linguists, philosophers, psychologists and sociologists but however one chooses to approach the issue, it is clear, as Shotter (1993) states, 'that, at least for some of us...identity has become the watchword of the times, for it provides the much needed vocabulary in terms of which we now define our loyalties and our commitments'.

Most contemporary writers reject any notion of fixed identity or personality: the prevailing theme is of the social construction of identity (Giddens, 1991; Shotter, 1993; Widdicombe and Wooffitt, 1995). The social model of self rejects ideas of innate personality, or of a self fixed solely through childhood socialization and experience. Throughout all the different theoretical positions held by interactionists like Goffman (1959), ethnomethodologists like Garfinkel (1967), labelling theorists like Lemert (1972), social constructionists like Berger and Luckman (1967), construct theorists like Kelly (1955) or the various post-structuralist, post-modernist theorists like Harré (1979), Foucault (1988) and Shotter (1984), there is broadly speaking, a common model of the person, a model epitomized in this quotation:

> Everyday life is, above all, life with and by means of the language I share with my fellowmen [sic].... What is more, I hear myself as I speak: my own subjective meanings are made objectively and continuously available to me and *ipso facto* become 'more real' to me... I objectivate my own being by means of language....
>
> *Berger and Luckman, 1966*

The social self, therefore, is a conception of the person as a being whose identity is continuously shaped by experience and who is affirmed or altered by interaction with other people. Though each approach differs in the extent to which this social self is determined by the power wielded by others or the dominant discourses of a society, all accept to some degree the idea of the self as something constructed from everyday experience and thus potentially open to change. Each approach differs in the extent to which language structures or reflects reality but all assign it a critical role. For it is language, either in the sense that it moulds thought internally or reflects the external attributions which others attach to a person, which mediates a person's identity. Whether language shapes or reflects the personal conception of self or the social labels that other people use, ultimately it either establishes and organizes the identity or communicates it.

In its simplest form identity may be understood as an interaction between the individual self-conception and the conception held of that person by others. It involves two essential questions, 'Who am I?' and 'Where do I belong?' Though it is possible to attempt to answer these questions solely at the personal level, this is an unsatisfactory approach because it ignores the extent to which individuals construct their personal identity through membership of different social and ethnic groups and through membership of particular societies, and also ignores the role of other people in categorizing or stereotyping individuals as being in or from particular groups. Answering the question 'Who am I?' may begin with an identification of personal characteristics such as height, weight, hair colour and traits such as honesty, reliability and intelligence, but it is apparent that such differentiation cannot take place in a social vacuum. It involves a more or less explicit comparison with other individuals or groups; taller than whom, more reliable than whom? At some point identification involves the question of ethnicity and group membership. Both Volosinov and Billig make this point. 'Any instance of self-awareness... is an act of gauging oneself against some social norm. Social evaluation is, so to speak, the socialization of oneself and one's behaviour. In becoming aware of myself, I attempt to look at myself, as it were through the eyes of another' (Volosinov, 1976). Similarly, Billig (1976) states that 'one does not identify *per se*, but one has to identify with something or someone'. He notes that identification with a social group is a complex two-way process, in which one is acted upon and in turn acts upon others. Because personal and group identification takes place within specific historical and social contexts, it is therefore fluid and open to change arising from events external to the individual/group, as well as from events and ideas originating within them. Recognition of both these critical elements avoids an overly deterministic approach to individual self-concept while still acknowledging the significance of external factors such as disadvantage and discrimination.

LANGUAGE AND IDENTITY

Language is a crucial factor in the processes of identification through the actual words used to express identity, such as 'black', 'Serbian', 'woman', and through the use of particular forms or types of language, where the medium itself rather than the content is the message. When words like 'black' are used, it is frequently assumed that all people thus categorized have a common characteristic, typically that they are non-white, or that they share similar experiences of discrimination, or that they share a common political perception of their social position (Mama, 1992). Such typifications which may help us make sense of the world by simplifying the complex reality carry certain dangers within them, especially when, as Thompson (1993) observes, 'we refuse to let logic or evidence challenge' them.

The role of stereotypes in promoting and maintaining discrimination and oppression has been widely noted. When we use words to categorize the world we may erroneously assume that the words represent some objective reality. This assumption, elevated in the 17th century to a philosophical doctrine by John Locke who believed words were the 'nominal essences' of the real world, continues to bedevil our thinking. As we have seen in Chapter 1, words are social creations not natural facts; one consequence of assuming that words are direct representations of a fixed reality is an overemphasis upon the common features of groups, that is, on their supposed similarities. For example, Castex (1994) has shown how the presumption of a common Spanish culture indicated by the terms 'Hispanic' and 'Latino' in the USA is mistaken. Hispanics, according to the Federal Government's definition of the term, actually originate from 25 different nations and speak a significant number of languages other than Spanish – for example, English, Dutch, French and numerous native American languages such as Quechua and Guaraní. For many Hispanics, Spanish is only their second language.

Billig (1976) has pointed out the 'dual nature of categorization', emphasizing that the process is not simply about the supposed similarities between people in the identified category, but about differentiation from other people who are not. This aspect of identification may be overlooked when attempting to understand how and why individuals and groups define themselves in particular ways. Understanding the process of identification of people into groups, whether done by themselves or others, necessitates a recognition of this duality, of the supposed similarities of group members, together with the supposed differences between them and others outside of it.

TWO EXAMPLES OF LANGUAGE TRANSFORMATION

The following examples illustrate the role of language in the process of establishing or confirming group identity. Each case also indicates the dual nature of categorization as a two-way process in which people identify similarities between themselves and others within the group, and perceive difference between the group and outsiders.

The first example is that of black youngsters of West Indian origin born in Britain. While black people have been present in Britain since Roman times, numbers were always small and, though the majority of the present black population originate from post-war migration, even today they only comprise approximately 5% of the total population. After the Second World War, immigrants were encouraged by successive governments who sought their labour to promote and sustain the post-war economic boom. Because most young black people growing up in the 1960s and 1970s, were the first members of their families to be born in Britain, their experience of life was in several critical respects different from that of their parents.

Many of their parents could be characterized as skilled working class. They had trained as electricians, nurses, carpenters, and so on, but upon arrival were rarely able to secure employment commensurate with their qualifications and experience. Like many immigrants into Britain they were treated as a reserve labour force and had little option but to take the most menial and low-paid jobs in order to survive. Their initial hopes and aspirations of a better life in Britain were thwarted and many were shocked by the increasingly overt racism which faced them. The superficial egalitarianism of the war years, when many had served in Britain's armed forces, quickly evaporated as West Indians replaced the Irish at the bottom of Britain's hierarchical and racist society. Research on their response to this unhappy situation is patchy; what is clear, however, is that it was not, for the most part, political. For many people religion provided solace and a sense of community as well as the promise of better things to come. Others, as Norman (1985) has described, viewed their stay in Britain as a temporary one and so coped with discrimination and disadvantage in the comforting belief that they would eventually return home to the Caribbean. However, in the absence of much substantive research into the political response to discrimination, we should avoid any stereotypical portrayal of 'West Indian immigrants as acquiescent, stoical and uncomplaining' as this ignores the 'many individuals who, from the earliest days of migration, openly questioned the justice of the treatment of black people' (Edwards, 1986).

Their children's experience differed most in one important respect – home for them was not a West Indian island, but British cities like Birmingham, Cardiff, London and Manchester. Their lives began in Britain and, throughout their childhood, their parents' aspirations for them focused upon education and getting a good job. The old accents, dialects and patois of the West Indies were often perceived by them and their parents as unsophisticated and a sign of poor education. This was reinforced by the attitudes of many educationalists, some of whom misunderstood Bernstein's work on speech codes and therefore, from the best of motives, misguidedly sought to improve the educational chances of black children by changing their language. Others clearly espoused overtly racist attitudes towards Creole and patois, which was variously described as 'babyish', 'very relaxed, like the way they walk' and as 'plantation English which is socially unacceptable and inadequate for communication' (Edwards, 1986). Most black children born in Britain learnt or assumed the accents and language of their white contemporaries, or sometimes aspired to an American black vernacular copied from their heroes in popular music.

By the end of the 1960s Britain's economy was in trouble and black workers and school-leavers, like reserve labour forces everywhere, were being squeezed out of employment or were unable to get jobs in the first place. The disillusionment was rapid but was not generally politicized in terms of social action, but was expressed in a growing disaffection with life in Britain (Hiro, 1973; Ely and Denney, 1987). The racism experienced more generally was now compounded by poverty and unemployment. Hebdige (1975) and other writers

(Cashmore and Troyna, 1982) have argued that interest in Rastafarianism and a re-evaluation of West Indian music such as ska, bluebeat and later reggae, grew in response to the increasing sense of alienation. 'Some rude boys began to grow the dreadlocks and many took to wearing woollen stocking caps, often in the green, gold and red of the Ethiopian flag to proclaim their alienation from the west...' (Hebdige, 1975). Hebdige has argued that music, dress, language and belief were critical elements 'used by young blacks to transmute a situation of extreme cultural dependence into one of virtual autonomy'. The adoption of Jamaican patois and the development of Rastafarian speech forms such as 'I and I' in place of 'You and me', by many young black people was a conscious means of rejecting the derogation of racism, the linguistic switch becoming a means of resisting the ideology of assimilation, and allowing the assertion of a different and more positive identity (Hebdige, 1975). This transformation of language can be seen a form of symbolic reversal, in that it explicitly rejected the formerly accepted speech codes in favour of language that not only asserted a new identity but could be used to reject and exclude white values and people. Minority language speakers with little effective power may use language as a protest, not simply through its content but by switching the form or type of language as a dissociative measure (Giles *et al.*, 1977).

From my own experience working in residential child care in the early 1970s, the transformation was rapid and effective. Within a few months black teenagers switched speech patterns and adopted new linguistic codes. Language, dress and music became clear symbols of a changing identity. The relatively few children in care who originated directly from the Caribbean, and who had hitherto been viewed by the British-born children as crude and unsophisticated, became role models in the new order. In my own workplace these changes were generally viewed unfavourably by white and black staff alike, which of course served to reaffirm for many children the desirability of the new identity. From my own observations, I saw that these changes quickly helped many children become more self-confident and assertive and less confused; they had consciously or unconsciously realized that they did not have to 'fit in', that they could choose to be different.

Edwards's study *Language in a Black Community* (Edwards, 1986) affirms the continuing importance of patois to black youngsters – levels of use and awareness of the symbolic functions of language-switching remain high. Patois continues to be widely used to mark ethnic identity and to express opposition and rejection to imposed values, but its use is not always overtly intended in these ways: sometimes usage is simply an act of accommodation, that is, of fitting in with the prevailing social context.

The second example of how a marginalized group may change or affirm their identity in response to their position within the wider society is drawn from the experience of the Welsh. Historically they are a people squeezed by invasion and economic domination into the western fringes of mainland Britain. They are the survivors of the original Britons, speaking a language derived from

Brythonic and, like many small nations, the Welsh have had to define and rede-fine themselves in response to the actions of other, more powerful people (Pugh, 1994a, b; Williams, 1985). Resistance to perceived oppression has at times been fierce, with extensive and prolonged strikes, rioting, demonstration and sabotage (Williams, 1988a). Wales continues to be one of the most economically deprived areas of Britain, with high levels of unemployment and relatively low wage rates.

For many years the Welsh language was suppressed by legislation, by delib-erate omission and by a cultural hegemony so successful that speaking Welsh was thought by many to be unsophisticated and a sign of poor education (Pugh, 1994b). The shift to English brought with it the meanings embedded in the English language; the Welsh have been stereotyped and devalued. The verb 'welsh/welch' has become a synonym for cheating and evasion; in popular imagery the Welsh have been portrayed as shifty and untrustworthy. Consequently, successive generations of Welsh children have grown up either not learning their native language or being ashamed of speaking it. Two students whose first language is Welsh once described to me how they returned home from their first day at school speaking gobbledygook to each other. When asked by their parents what they were doing they replied that they were speak-ing English! Clearly, these students had already learnt a damaging lesson at school about the value of their own language compared to English.

Today around 20% of the total population of Wales speak Welsh, but in the two northernmost counties it rises to over 30%, with rates as high as 85% in some localities (1991 Census). However, the Welsh Social Survey (Welsh Office, 1992) revealed that 32.4% of children aged 3–15 years are Welsh-speak-ing. This rising proportion indicates the increasing value attached to learning the Welsh language, which is now actively promoted within some school districts. Similarly, there is also an increasing number of adult learners. In Wales the improved status of the language, arising from political and cultural activism, together with its re-emergence in education, business and government, has led to generation gaps within families in terms of the ability to speak Welsh. Grandparents may speak Welsh because they learned it through common usage, children may learn it at school but their parents may have only a shaky grasp of it because it was not the *lingua franca* when they were young nor were they taught it at school. Sympathy for Cymdeithas yr Iaith Gymraeg/Welsh Language Movement among working-class people, who once viewed it as an organization of middle-class educated literary activists with whom they had little in common, increased throughout the 1980s. The positive representation of Welshness on the TV channel S4C, and in the Welsh media generally, support a more distinctive group identification. The growing use of the written language is being used to develop an explicitly feminist Welsh identity for women (Aaron *et al.*, 1994), and Urdd, the Welsh Youth movement, has over 50 000 members. The positive mood is also seen in the conscious adoption of Welsh names for a whole range of groups and organizations from housing associations and charities to rock bands, dance groups and business enterprises. However, while Cymdeithas yr Iaith and Urdd have stressed the unique elements of Welsh culture, the more recent identification of community, though based upon a perception of commonality, also owes much to the increasingly popular rejection of Englishness. That is, it relies as much upon differentiation/dissociation as upon identification/association.

Thus the Welsh language has become a 'rallying point for ethnic identity' (Edwards, 1977) among a group that perceives itself to be under pressure; to define oneself as Welsh has become as much a statement of being non-English as a statement of adherence to a common culture. The Welsh language has been both the subject and the means of protest at English domination. This is reflected in the voting patterns for the different political parties over the past 15 years. If the increasing acceptance and use of Welsh language were simply about the language and Welsh culture then one might have expected the nationalist party, Plaid Cymru, to have gained most of the votes at the expense of the ruling Conservative Party, but it is the Labour Party who have remained the main party of opposition. It could be, as Borland, Fevre and Denney (1992) imply, that the relative success/failure of the parties reflects the extent to which each organization embraces particular conceptions of community. For example, the identification of the nationalists with Welsh language and an exclusive notion of community might prove unattractive for the majority of Welsh people, whose first language is English. The increasing use of Welsh, particularly among young people, obviously does reflect some sense of uniqueness and commonality, together with the recognition that what was once a barrier to employment and promotion may now be an asset, but it arguably also reflects an increasing alienation from the political and economic consequences of life under English Conservative government.

Though the specific features of the experience of young black and Welsh people are markedly different, their reaction to their economic and social position has in some respects been similar, that is, to invest significance in their respective languages. Both groups shared a feeling of being non-English and being thought inferior and both have sought positive validation of their position through a conscious transformation of language and dialect. In Wales, this is most marked in the north and is indicated by both the choice of language and by its content. For example, phrases from colonial Africa like 'white settlers' have been used to describe English incomers to the region. Many black youngsters lacking a formal alternative language adapted and developed the patois of their parents and grandparents in order to affirm their new identity and reject the assimilationist assumptions made by successive British governments, and originally accepted by some of their parents. Superficially, the position of black youngsters appears to differ from their Welsh counterparts in so far as there may appear to be a discontinuity between their experiences and those of their parents. However, we should be wary of overemphasizing this; as Edwards (1992) notes, 'Both generations share many common values and cultural experiences. For example, a significant minority of young British Black people attend church and conform closely to parental expectations of how they should behave.' Perhaps the greatest differences between the reactions of black and Welsh young people derive from the individual experience of racism, which arguably impacts more upon everyday personal experience, and from the explicit politicization of language and the relative success of social action within Wales. There are relatively few formal channels of protest available for black young people; thus the significance of language as both an associative and a dissociative measure is exemplified today by the popularity of rap music, whose powerful attraction derives in part from its language, which is often deliberately provocative and intended as a form of protest.

GROUP AND PERSONAL IDENTITY IN SITUATIONS OF DISADVANTAGE

The ways in which minority groups think of themselves will vary according to their perception of their position relative to the majority or dominant groups within a society. Tajfel (1974, 1978) has proposed that members of a minority group, that is, one that is inferior in terms of status or power in a particular society, can either accept or reject their position. If they accept the prevailing definition there are two ways in which they can attempt to achieve a more positive self-image; both are individualistic strategies. The first is to compare themselves favourably with other members of their own group, that is, to restrict the frame of reference. Coates (1993) has suggested that, although women have begun to think of themselves differently, many of them still compare themselves with other women in areas such as personal appearance, cookery and child-care. The second is to attempt to join the superior group. This option is obviously limited by the extent to which a person can pass as a member of the more dominant group.

The concept of **passing** is most well known from Goffman's (1968) work on stigma, in which he suggests that, if a person has an identity that is discreditable but is not yet discredited – that is, there is something about them that could be stigmatized and would be viewed negatively by others if it were known, then there are several coping strategies that they may adopt to deal with this situation. Passing is therefore the third stage of reaction to stigmatization, the first being when the person learns what the 'normal' point of view is, the second when the person becomes aware that they are 'disqualified' according to it and the third, which includes passing, is learning to cope. Passing is therefore one of the coping strategies that a potentially discreditable person may use to deal with situations where they know or strongly suspect that other people will devalue them if the fact of their difference became known. Passing means to present oneself as 'normal' by deliberately disguising or hiding the potentially discrediting feature. Thus someone whose spoken English is heavily accented, in a manner which they feel others will perceive negatively, may choose to disguise their voice by modulating their tone and pronunciation or by avoiding speech altogether and using written communication instead. As in instances of people with HIV and AIDS, this type of 'control of identity information' (Goffman, 1968) has great significance for relationships with professional helpers and friends, who may be 'wise' as to what the passer wishes to conceal. The professional principle of confidentiality can be seen as one response to this type of privileged knowledge. For members of 'discreditable' groups, passing strategies commonly exact a toll in stress and anxiety upon the passer, who may completely alter, control and regulate their everyday life in order to maintain the appearance of 'normality'.

Whether an individual feels any need to adopt coping strategies depends upon the visibility and obtrusiveness of their difference. The extent of visibility depends upon whether the difference is one that can readily be perceived by others, whereas obtrusiveness refers to the extent that the difference gets in the way of communication with others. The fact that a person has had a colostomy, for example, is not usually visible to other people so it is relatively easy for such a person to appear 'normal' in most situations without it becoming apparent. In contrast, a person with a speech impediment can only disguise their difficulty until they are faced with situations where speech is required. Even when the fact that a person has had a colostomy is known, it still does not usually obtrude into the situation in the same way that a speech impediment does. There are of course many situations in which people who may be disadvantaged and discriminated against have little opportunity to pass. This is frequently true for people whose appearance conveys the potentially discriminating fact about them, for most black people, wheelchair users and women these facts are nearly always present in their interactions with others.

Returning to Tajfel's typification of minority group reactions, where individuals and groups accept the dominant definition of inferiority, there is arguably a third possibility. This is, that individuals within the group may internalize the negative definition within a self-conception of low worth and esteem. For example, as Finkelstein and French (1993) have noted, if people with disabilities 'think of themselves in the same way as able-bodied people think of them and behave as others expect them to... the self-fulfilling prophecy... it is hardly surprising, therefore [that this] sometimes leads to depression, passivity, anxiety and hopelessness... which in turn may lead able-bodied people to regard them as unmotivated and poorly adjusted'. Maxime (1986) has illustrated the consequences of internalization of negative self-worth. She has described the difficulties and problems of a young black boy who initially denied the fact of his blackness and thought of himself as white. In the USA this question of black identity has received much more attention and there are a number of black identity development models, the most well known being the work of Cross (1971, 1978) and Jackson (1975). In both models there is a recognition that it is difficult, if not impossible, to establish a sustainable positive identity in a racist society, without moving from a white frame of reference for comparison to a black one. The individual who internalizes the prevailing racist definitions may never achieve this. Consequently, her/his personal moods and reactions should be interpreted within the social context rather than within a narrow psychological one. However, we should remember that internalization of negative esteem is only one possibility and note that it is by no means inevitable.

Owusu-Bempah (1994) has criticized the tendency of white workers to assume the prevalence of poor self-concept among black people. He found that they used the assumption to pathologize black children. 'Clearly, the respondents saw the black children's friendship with white children as pathological, in spite of their "multi-racial" environment – their school'. In this instance, they believed that the black child's friendliness to white children was, in itself, evidence of poor self-concept! The harmful consequences of assuming the inevitability of poor self-concept are obvious – inappropriate and damaging interventions resulting from self-fulfilling assessments.

If individuals or groups reject or oppose the prevailing definition, that is, reject the inferior status, they may react in three possible ways.

- They may try to adopt the values of the superior/dominant group and try to gain equality with them without compromising their identity. Coates has noted that women who individually attempt to assimilate into the dominant group will adopt many male speech features such as lowering the tone of their voice; using taboo and swear words; becoming more assertive in group interaction; changing to falling intonation rather than rising intonation towards the end of sentences; switching the focus of their speech topics towards traditionally male ones, such as cars and sport; retaining those non-standard accents which have become more acceptable in business and politics, for example, Scottish and northern accents as opposed to Birmingham or Liverpool accents.
- They may seek to redefine what have previously been defined as negative characteristics, as demonstrated in the deliberate adoption of patois and Creole speech patterns by young black people in the earlier example. The shift in the 1960s from the use of the word 'coloured' to 'black' reflected more than positive appreciation of what had previously been seen as a negative characteristic, skin colour. It also indicated a shift in political awareness as it came to mean people affected by racism (Mama, 1992).
- They may create new dimensions for comparison, which will give value to previously unrecognized characteristics. This frequently involves creating new words or concepts to express the new or rediscovered abilities. As Coates has noted, it is likely that these last two strategies will occur together; thus the traditional stereotypical 'weak' qualities of women, such as sensitivity, non-violence and caring, become emphasized positively in contrast to the stereotypical 'strong' male qualities of assertiveness, competitiveness and aggression, which are devalued as divisive, violent and antisocial.

Tajfel suggests that these reactions tend to occur sequentially, and Coates in her review of the model's application to women also accepts this view. The typification of minority group response is relevant in the two examples described earlier. In the case of British-born black young people who rejected the prevailing definitions, they adopted two of these strategies – the symbolic reversal of negative characteristics and the creation of new dimensions for rating themselves. The example of the Welsh differs in that there is no clearly defined difference between generations, but it clearly illustrates the effects of the transformation of value in redefining Welshness, as indicated by the use of the Welsh language as a positive statement.

CONCLUSION

Within the helping professions an awareness that language is not simply about communication but is also a means of creating and asserting identity is likely to lead to a greater appreciation of its less obvious functions, particularly its crucial role in establishing personal and group identity. These identities are not fixed but are the product of a dialectic between individuals/groups and society; 'societies have histories in the course of which specific identities emerge; these histories are, however, made by men [*sic*] with specific identities' (Berger and Luckman, 1967). Models such as Tajfel's can help us to recognize the significance of language for disadvantaged people and groups, by highlighting some of the typical ways in which they may react to their situation. As we shall see in the discussion of language and power in Chapter 5, we should also be aware that when we are in positions of power, as in our professional roles, then we too may have many unmobilized assumptions about what is normal. In our work we may adopt slang and jargon, language which helps to define our professional identity, and unwittingly confuse or alienate our clients.

We should also remember the lesson to be drawn from the example of the psychiatric examination of the Asian woman in Chapter 1, that not only do the identities that we create and expect of others differ, but the 'Western conception of the person as... a distinctive whole... [is] a rather peculiar idea within the context of the world's cultures' (Geertz, cited in Widdicombe and Wooffitt, 1995) – peculiar, that is, in the stress that it places upon the separateness of the individual and the emphasis it places upon individual traits. Perhaps a more accurate rendering of the notion of identity is to understand it as a culturally specific creation which varies from one situation to another; this conception thus allows recognition of the multifaceted nature of our identities. Thus, when we behave and think differently in different circumstances, we are not acting falsely or denying some 'real' self, we are re-presenting and re-creating our ideas of who we think we are, and who we think other people are too.

4

Using language

Someone once... said that a fish would be the last to discover the existence of water.

Burgoon, Hunsaker and Dawson, 1994

INTRODUCTION

The quotation from Burgoon is used to illustrate how difficult it can be to see the most pervasive elements of our environment – communication and conversation are very much the taken-for-granted aspects of human behaviour. This chapter reviews the main ideas developed in the body of theory and research called conversation analysis, which attempts to discover and describe the unwritten and implicit 'rules' that underpin ordinary conversation. These 'rules' or orderly qualities concern how people convey and construe meaning, how they construct and act in conversation. The question of how we actually use language has been one of the central concerns of linguists. They have developed a wide range of approaches to explaining this – as we saw in Chapter 1, some have tried to identify the formal grammatical structures that underpin particular languages while others have attempted to describe other features which might apply universally. There are an enormous number of empirical studies which have investigated more narrowly focused linguistic features – such as phonology (patterns of sounds), phonetics (pronunciation), morphology (word structure) and lexicon (vocabulary) – with a few notable exceptions, these studies have not referred to broader issues of culture and power and are thus not directly relevant to the concerns of this book.

Governments have tried to prescribe which language should be used or have attempted to maintain the 'purity' of particular languages by formal declarations regarding the acceptability of various words and linguistic features. For example, in both France and Germany there are lists of approved names which must be used in order to confer legal identity upon a newborn child. However, the way in which we use language has not yet been satisfactorily captured by one explanation, nor has it always been subject to the prescriptions of govern-ment. Most of the 'top-down' explanations are open to the criticism of overdetermination (Spender, 1980), excessive reductionism (Chomsky, 1968) and overgeneralization (the behaviourist accounts). Despite their highly abstract conceptualizations, they tend to give precedence to one feature while ignoring the significance of others, to oversimplify the variability of language use and to provide an inadequate account of how language is used in every-day life.

In contrast to the grand theories of language promoted by writers like Chomsky, there are approaches which have tried to study language use empir-ically from the 'bottom up'. I have subsumed most of these under the general heading of conversation analysis, though there are writers who might usually be identified in different terms, such as communication theorists, network analysts and ethnomethodologists. Ethnographers, for example, have tried to identify and map the social and cultural factors that influence language use in particular social groups, while communication theorists have attempted to establish the factors that influence the effectiveness of communication. However, for the present, I shall use the term 'conversation analysis' as a collective term for these more empirical approaches, though, as Atkinson (1988) has pointed out, even within the subgroup of ethnomethodology there are considerable differences between writers. An erudite exploration of these particular differences can be found in Williams (1992); they are most marked in the differing epistemologies adopted by the different approaches; that is, the extent to which they think it is possible to **know** something, in the sense that something is perceived as true or real. Some writers, like the ethnomethodologist Garfinkel (1967), disavow any notion that there is a real objective world that we can discover, but accept that while all knowledge is relative, that is, located in particular times, people, and societies, it is never-theless possible to obtain more accurate and less distorted descriptions and theories of human action from the participants themselves.

The prefix *ethno*, from the Greek for 'a nation', indicates the general orientation of many of these approaches, which is a concern to understand a language and the social world of the people using it, to try to grasp something of the subjective appreciation that a native speaker has of her/his language and the society it represents. Unlike theorists who have focused upon formal and written language, most of these studies are concerned with an empirical examination of how people actually speak to each other. Though ethnogra-phy, ethnomethodology and some forms of communication theory originate from different intellectual traditions within anthropology, philosophy and psychology, to some degree they share a common focus upon the following:

- the subjectivity of meaning;
- the construction of the 'common sense';

- the 'rules' or conventions of conversation;
- the idea of social role;
- conversational competence and linguistic repertoire.

These approaches have provided valuable description and useful analytical concepts which aid our understanding of how we use language, although, as will become apparent later, there are some difficulties with these approaches, especially the tendency to omit issues of power.

THE SUBJECTIVITY OF MEANING

In their studies of so-called primitive societies anthropologists quickly came to realize that much of the behaviour they witnessed could not be understood from their Western point of view: much of it initially seemed to them to be weird, irrational and unproductive. However, they realized that it clearly had significance for those who engaged in it and that unless anthropologists attempted to grasp the meaning the participants attached to the behaviour, they would continue to misunderstand or misinterpret it. Within sociology, a similar awareness of the importance of understanding subjective meaning was developed in the work of Weber (Freund, 1968), who used the word *verstehen* to indicate the necessity of understanding the actor's point of view and of the importance of the sociologist reflecting upon the nature of her/his own consciousness. From philosophy too, in the work of the phenomenologists Husserl (1970) and Schutz (1972), there has been a challenge to the positivistic conception of the world as a fixed and objective reality governed by natural laws.

This emphasis upon subjectivity was also prominent in the work of antipsychiatric writers like Laing (1969, Laing and Esterson, 1970) and Szasz (1972), who argued that madness could be seen as a rational response to an illogical situation, or that the patient was in some sense the victim of events whose causes lay beyond her/his control. This perspective is clearly seen in the following quotation: 'What we are setting out to do is to show that Maya's experiences and actions, especially those deemed most schizophrenic, become intelligible as they are seen in the light of her family situation. This situation is not only the family seen from without, but the family as experienced by each of its members from inside' (Laing and Esterson, 1970).

Whatever the merits and demerits of their theories, their impact lay in the manner in which they de-pathologized the deviant person and affirmed the importance of understanding disorder from an interactionist perspective. They recognized that the causes of pathology often lay outside the individual and not within her/him. Thus, even the strangest of behaviours might be open to some degree of understanding, that sometimes bizarre language and meaning might be rendered intelligible.

Conversation analysis has also focused upon people who are different or 'deviant' in some way and has attempted to show how apparently illogical actions might be reinterpreted as rational once the participant's language and meaning were appreciated (Becker, 1963). The term 'deviant' was used by many writers not as a moralistic judgement about people but as a way of describing people who were outsiders on the margins of society. Within coun-selling and social work this approach has been institutionalized in the practice rule – that all interventions should begin from where the client is, not from where the worker thinks s/he should be – that is, to accept the reality of the subjective experience of others (Burnard 1989). This means one does not have to agree with it, nor reject it, but to recognize the significance of the client's subjective reality as the starting point for work with that person. For example, Kempe and Kempe (1978), writing on child abuse, identified four factors typi-cally associated with child abuse; among these was the presence of crisis. By this they meant a subjective crisis felt by the carer, a crisis defined in the client's terms, not the doctor's or social worker's. The risks of not properly 'hearing' and recognizing the significance of the felt experience of a parent under stress have, unfortunately, become apparent as successive inquiries into child deaths have shown.

The linguistic studies undertaken by Garfinkel (1967), Gumperz and Hymes (Gumperz, 1982b, Gumperz and Hymes, 1972, Hymes, 1977) and the sociologi-cal and psychological studies of interaction undertaken by Goffman (1974), Cicourel (1973) and others all put the question of meaning at the forefront of their work. Typically, they describe the meanings that underpin everyday conversation and behaviour by showing how meaning is determined by both the words and the social context. One common thread has been to establish what Schutz termed the 'stock knowledge at hand' used to make sense of conversa-tions that otherwise might seem confusing and chaotic. Heritage (1984) demon-strates this in the following example of conversation:

A. I have a fourteen year old son.

B. Well, that's all right.

A. I also have a dog.

B. Oh, I'm sorry.

This only becomes intelligible when we understand the context, which is a conversation between a prospective tenant and a landlord. Hartley (1993) provides a good example of how ambiguous even apparently mundane state-ments can be. If the morning after a party, your neighbour asks you the question 'Did you have a good time last night?', there are at least four possible interpre-tations of what this might mean:

● Is it a genuine query, or a cynical attempt to soften you up, so that s/he may borrow something from you?

- Is it a subtle accusation about any noise or disturbance you may have made?
- Is it designed to make you feel uncomfortable because you did not invite him?
- Is it an expression of his loneliness?

A decision on what is meant will depend upon a number of factors, including the tone of voice, the intonation, the history of interaction with the neighbour, the non-verbal communication and so on. What is notable is that very quickly you would be able to establish what is meant by the question, either by guessing it correctly first time, or by establishing which other meaning is intended from subsequent conversation. Hartley (1993) provides another striking example of how meaning is contextualized by other information, by citing a newspaper headline from 1943 which baldly stated '8th Army Push Bottles Up Jerries'. The intended meaning derived from the fact that there was a war going on, but out of the immediate context of time and place, the possibly comic misreading is obvious.

THE CONSTRUCTION OF 'COMMON SENSE'

Recognition of the subjectivity of meaning led logically to an examination of how meaning was established, maintained and altered. Conversation analysis has shown that meanings are not fixed entities, but are dynamic and vary according to person, time and place. Thus, it is proposed, we are all engaged in a more or less continuous process of constructing and reconstructing meaning through our interaction with other people. It is accepted that some meanings are more stable than others, but this stability is not thought to originate from outside the participants in conversation, but to be established by them through repetition and reconfirmation. Consequently, there has been a particular focus upon the **common sense** that is established between individuals and within social groups, and especially upon the informal nature of the processes involved. Some of this common sense is widely shared, but much of it is specific to particular groups. Garfinkel (1967) sought to establish the significance of this taken for granted knowledge and to demonstrate the far-reaching extent of it.

The existence of this common sense can be revealed in many ways: through observation of children's learning of language, through social dislocation when people are out of their normal context, and through analysis of how conversationalists deal with changes in circumstances that lie beyond their control. On a summer camping trip many years ago, I remember asking a young boy to put the milk into a bucket of water and being dismayed at seeing him take the top off the bottle and pour the contents into the bucket! Such literal reading of language shows that meaning may depend upon other understandings which predate the conversation. In fact, in some forms of mental illness it is precisely this type of literalness which is taken as an indicator of cognitive disorder. Note that it is taken as a symptom of illness not misunderstanding! The perils of assuming a universal common sense were noted in Chapter 1, in regard to Gumperz's observation that misunderstandings were more likely to happen when people thought they were alike than when they perceived obvious difference between them.

Common sense can be established and negotiated in subtle ways which are not always immediately apparent from a literal reading of conversation. The implicit nature of many understandings is often only indirectly alluded to – they are easily missed until the listener becomes attuned to the commonalities and the possibilities which may develop during the conversation. This pre-knowledge not only allows conversationalists to contextualize information, it also enables them to fill in gaps in what is being said. This skill is often highly developed among some people with partial hearing loss who, through the use of pre-existing knowledge and awareness of possible conversational options, become adept at filling in the gaps in conversations. Most of us have probably experienced the embarrassment of misreading a conversation and misunderstanding the other person's meanings. Crystal (1987) has noted how comedy often relies upon our awareness of the conventions that structure and aid our understandings of discourse. We understand and make sense of the one-sided conversations of comedians, like Bob Newhart in his tobacco or driving instructor routines, because we are able to 'fill in the gaps', by imagining what the other person's responses are.

The professional dangers of assuming a common sense with other professionals has been most starkly demonstrated by the frequency of misunderstanding revealed in child abuse inquiries. For example, the assumption that another professional's visit to a child's home automatically meant that the child had been directly observed, has on at least two occasions proved to be tragically mistaken.

THE 'RULES' OF CONVERSATION

Analysis of actual conversation reveals that much of it is ungrammatical (by the standards of written language – see Chapter 1), unfinished and replete with hesitation and apparent uncertainty. This lack of structure is more apparent than real, in fact, there are many unwritten rules and rituals which govern our spoken interactions and help us to make sense of them (Sacks and Shegloff, 1973). While we are aware of some general rules, such as when to look at people when talking and when not to, the conventions are often tacit. For example: 'Routines for concluding a conversation are particularly complex, and cooperation is crucial if it is not to end abruptly, or in an embarrassed silence.... A widespread convention is for visitors to say they must leave sometime before they actually intend to depart, and for the hosts to ignore the remark. The second mention then permits both parties to act' (Crystal, 1987).

Of course some conventions are represented by changes in the formal structure of a language. As Romaine (1994) has noted, social distinctions are marked by grammar and vocabulary in many languages such as Japanese, Spanish and Welsh, where the different modes of address indicate different degrees of status and formality. While many of the 'rules' in English are much less formal, they are nevertheless present – Romaine observes that 'speakers of American English offer each other more compliments than do English speakers in South Africa', and interestingly are taught to accept them more. Furthermore, compliments from women are less likely to be 'accepted with simple thanks by both men and women'. There are tacit 'rules' for 'turn-taking', which indicate when to interrupt and when to speak, which are more complex than simply knowing when to butt in – for example, the recognition of clues given by a speaker that signal a willingness to give way to another speaker. Different ethnic groups can have different rules for turn-taking; in some societies it is the oldest person who takes precedence in conversation, while in others it is men. As we shall see in the next chapter, it is probable that power is a critical factor determining these variations and it may account for the reported differences between men's and women's turn-taking behaviour.

SOCIAL ROLE

Role playing is another aspect of conversational interaction that has been widely noted. The concept of role has been widely used to describe the idea that there are patterns of expectation or ways of behaving which vary according to a person's age, gender, occupation and relationship to others, and so on. Goffman did much to popularize the concept, suggesting that we are all actors with social roles to play, according to the situations and circumstances in which we find ourselves. When he applied this dramaturgical model to an analysis of the institutional life of a mental asylum he sceptically concluded that 'inmates and lower level staff are involved in a vast supportive action – an elaborate dramatized tribute – that has the effect, if not the purpose, of affirming that a medical like service is in progress here and that the psychiatric staff is providing it' (Goffman, 1961).

Furthermore, all roles are social because they operate in relation to the roles played by other people. Dahrendorf (1973) suggested that there were three levels of obligation in regard to any role:

- the things we must do;
- the things we should do;
- the things we can do.

The first level refers to absolute expectations, the second to what is usually done and the third to what is optional or potentially available for the role-player. Though Dahrendorf does imply some degree of choice, this conception of the person as an actor who assumes different roles that are pre-existing and prescribed has been criticized for painting an overly deterministic picture of human behaviour. The fundamental objection is that people do have some freedom of choice and roles do change, otherwise society would remain static. Most conversation analysts would reject an overly rigid conceptualization of role, but they do employ the concept because it provides a vital key to understanding how social stability is maintained. Thus, 'social roles are one feature of the manner in which social structure is mutually produced by actors as a feature of everyday activity such that social order is constantly created and recreated' (Williams, 1992). As we shall see in Chapter 5, the question of how free we are to change our behaviour and our ideas is central to the discussion on the relationship of language to power.

Nevertheless, the concept of roles has some utility, providing we do not assume their inevitability or rigidity. It is useful for understanding the expectations that we have of other people and ourselves, and especially in identifying the types of ideas and behaviour that people embrace. Goffman's (1968) work on stigmatized roles described the role options open to people who had some feature that was viewed negatively. The 'discreditable' feature might be some illness, disability, criminal record or sexual preference, but in each instance public knowledge of the feature would normally have damaging consequences for the person and their sense of self. The damaging consequences of such spoiled identities depends upon the extent to which the potentially stigmatized person accepts or rejects the negative identity, and the extent to which they can control personal information about their 'stigma' and perhaps pass as 'normal' (see the discussion of passing in Chapter 3). A fuller account of the nature of the relationship between role and identity is complex and beyond the intended scope of this book; however, for the interested reader, there is an interesting analysis of some of the theoretical problems in Widdicombe and Wooffitt, 1995. Goffman's analysis of the role of professionals, who are often 'wise' to a person's secret condition, remains a perceptive account of the collaborative aspects of the helping role.

Another interesting study of dramaturgical role in health professions was undertaken by Henslin and Briggs (1971), who looked at the language and interaction surrounding gynaecological examinations. These examinations of women, typically by male doctors, were found to be highly structured in ways that allowed the doctor and the patient to assume depersonalized, desexualized roles, with the female nurse acting as a confidante and collaborator to the patient. The doctors typically avoided eye contact with the patient and restricted conversation to specific medical issues. The patients, for the purpose of the examination, became non-persons who spoke little and moved only upon request. After the examination, when patients were dressed, consultations proceeded and patients resumed the role of responsible adult. Conversational roles may be less obvious than these examples. Berne (1968) has described many conversational strategies and gambits that may be used to channel the other speaker's contribution, leaving them with few options as to how they might respond.

Role theory was not intended by Goffman to provide an account of power and social action: he set out to describe and analyse face-to-face interaction and the strategies of self-presentation used to maintain the social self. His contention – that human interaction is a moral enterprise, in the sense that humans are continuously striving to present certain ideas about themselves and about other people, that is, to establish their preferred world-view – provides a useful account of the interplay of these differing conceptions, though, clearly, the obvious weakness of his approach lies in the absence of any explicit theory of power.

LINGUISTIC REPERTOIRE AND COMMUNICATIVE COMPETENCE

The term **communicative competence** has been used to distinguish the overall set of skills and knowledge used in conversation from the narrowly defined rules of written grammar (Hymes, 1972). While most writers, like Gumperz and Hymes (1972), use the term in a rather more restricted sense, to refer to the tacit understandings which structure meaning within conversations, I have used the term more broadly to refer also to the notion of linguistic repertoire. Conversational analysis has revealed that much of what was previously thought unremarkable and taken for granted is highly sophisticated and complex. A knowledge of conversational rules, strategies and context has been shown to be essential to the linguistic repertoire of a competent communicator. This competence embraces knowledge of a linguistic repertoire that includes turn-taking, bargaining and negotiation and so on. The following subsections describe some of the most important aspects of repertoire, such as code switching, accommodation and stereotyping.

Code switching

An essential aspect of linguistic repertoire is the ability to use different forms of language. For example, most bilingual speakers are aware of conventions determining when it is appropriate to switch from one language to another (Fishman, 1972), but even within a single language there are conventions about the appropriate register to use. In this context the term **register** is used to denote the different varieties of a language, such as legal, scientific or computer-speak which have developed in particular domains; slang and jargon can also be described as registers of speech. The term **code** is generally used to denote different formal systems of communication, such as different oral languages like English and Welsh, but also for different systems of language such as Morse Code, Seaspeak, Citizen's Band radio-speak and so on. Although 'code' is normally used as a general term encompassing all languages and 'register' is sometimes used for varieties within a single language, confusion arises because some writers use the terms interchangeably, while others use 'code' to refer to both. I have adopted the latter convention. The significance of the distinction for communicative competence arises from recognition of the capacity of competent speakers to switch codes, that is to switch from one language to another, or from one form to another.

Some social work students whose first language is Welsh and who are accustomed to using it mainly in the more informal domains of their lives have noted that, in situations where they are required to act with authority and speak more formally, such as in Court or in case conference, they felt their spoken Welsh was inadequate for the task. Whether this is objectively the case is not certain, but what is clear is that their ability to switch codes may have been hindered as much by a lack of confidence as by any lack of skill. It shows how the historical derogation and suppression of minority languages may affect individual performance long after the more repressive events have passed.

Code switching has various forms and signifies different things to different people. Trudgill (1983) has reported the research of David Parkin in Uganda, who described a situation where there were many different ethnic groups and languages spoken and it was common for people to speak two or three languages, such as English, Luganda (a local Bantu language) and Swahili. Conversation switched from one language to another according to the topic and the feelings being expressed. For example, two Kenyan exiles might use Swahili for demonstrating common feelings such as commiseration, whereas in a more competitive situation one speaker might initiate a switch to English, which both would perceive as less personal and intimate. Code switching, as shown by the examples of patois and Welsh in Chapter 3, can be used as a dissociative measure. In both instances, people consciously altered their choice of language and thus increased the difference between themselves and other people, in response to their perceived marginalization and as a means of affirming their group identity.

Rapid switching between language forms or types is called **language mixing** and may be used in a variety of ways, to demonstrate acceptance, disagreement, knowledge of other people, to emphasize a point, to use a more precise word and to humorous effect. It is commonly observed among bilingual speakers, who, as well as using it to express solidarity, may switch when they are tired or distracted, or use it to signal their attitudes towards the particular topic of conversation. Gumperz (1970) describes a situation in which two first-language Spanish speakers mixed Spanish and English during a discussion of smoking. English was used for more detached statements while Spanish was used to express the smoker's personal embarrassment at admitting the habit. In the case of social workers, lawyers, doctors and nurses, code switching and mixing can be used to demonstrate professional competency in formal settings. Alternatively, it may be used to demonstrate intimacy or friendliness, to be clear and unambiguous or, as in the case of slang and jargon, to emphasize identity and group cohesion. Edwards (1986) notes how the use of patois by some white people, a practice rejected by many young black people, is sometimes accepted as a marker of friendship and identification.

Linguistic accommodation

Accommodation refers to the process whereby speakers alter their language to become more like the person they are speaking to. Most people are aware that they do this consciously when speaking to different people, though this may also be an unconscious accommodation to another person. Linguists have long recognized this tendency for speakers to adjust their speech styles and language (Coupland and Giles, 1988). The main forms of such adjustments are towards convergence, that is when each speaker's language tends to become more like the other's, or towards divergence, that is, when they become less like each other. Accommodation may take the form of code switching or may be less dramatic. It may simply involve changes in intonation, pronunciation or vocabulary. As with code switching, there are many different reasons for this process: it may result from an awareness of another person's power, or from a desire to minimize difference from another person. Many people find that their accents become more like each other's when they converse. The process has even been noted among young children, who at the age of 12 months have been observed to produce deeper vocal sounds in the presence of their fathers than when with their mothers (Crystal, 1987).

Linguistic divergence may be indicated by code switching or differences of accent and syntax; its use may indicate dislike or disapproval or, as noted in the previous section, be an assertion of status difference or identity. The use of convergence and divergence is discussed further in Chapter 5.

Stereotyping

The question of the extent to which language reflects an external reality or shapes an internal one was a central issue in Chapter 1. I tentatively concluded that perhaps it does both, for we are presented with the world and language as other people use it, but we are each able to create our own meanings as well as reiterating those given to us. The words that we use can be seen as a shorthand way of communicating ideas, without having to explain exactly what we think they mean every time we use them; thus words can represent categories or generalizations of experience and meaning. For example, when we use the word 'car', we expect that other people will take this to mean a particular category of motor vehicle; although there are of course many varieties of motor car, which could be distinguished by colour, make, capacity, working order, ownership and so on, it is used in this reductive way because it is useful to do so. After all we do not wish to specify every detail each time we wish to make reference to a motor vehicle. In this case, the fact that the finer details get omitted is mostly irrelevant except when certain situations demand action, such as when we have to buy or sell a car or need to arrange motor insurance.

Unfortunately, the typification of people, their experiences and behaviour in simple word-terms can create as many problems as it solves. Problems arise when different people interpret words such as 'black' and its associated ideas and meanings differently. Furthermore, the typifications represented by particular words may not only become oversimplifications but end up bearing little relationship to the things they purport to represent. Stereotypes are typifications that have become embedded in our consciousness which may be inaccurate, biased and oversimplified and may be negative or positive in their connotations. The consequences of negative stereotypes of people were noted in Chapter 2 and are explored further in Chapter 5. It should be noted that stereotypes often persist despite contradictory evidence because they not only simplify the complexity of our social world but also serve important social and psychological functions for us. In this way stereotypes may contribute to the ideologies that legitimate existing forms of social behaviour. At their most benign they simplify complexity but at their most malign they derogate the real or supposed differences between people. The continuing use of stereotypes by individuals may indicate their economic, social, emotional or intellectual insecurity. It may also reveal strongly held ideological beliefs about society, beliefs which confer advantages on some people while disadvantaging others.

Communicative competence

As noted earlier, the term **communicative competence** is normally used in a more specific way than it is used within this chapter. The essence of this narrower idea is summarized by Crystal (1987), who described four maxims thought necessary for successful communication. These maxims or conventions have been derived from extensive observation of cooperative communicants, that is, from the speech of people who have been trying to 'get along with each other'. They are:

- the maxim of quality, which is that communicants should tell the truth or at least avoid wittingly giving inaccurate information;
- the maxim of quantity, which is that they should provide just enough information, not too much detail or too little;
- the maxim of relevance, which is that the information should relate to the topic at hand;
- the maxim of manner, which is that the speakers should provide their contributions in as orderly and unambiguous a fashion as possible.

However, the apparent simplicity of these maxims belies the immense complexity of our conversational behaviour. Widdicombe and Wooffitt (1995) refer to an example given by Sacks, in which a psychiatric social worker is talking to a suicidal patient. In the early part of the conversation the patient's previous interests and employment are discussed and he mentions that he was a hair stylist and 'did some fashions now and then, things like that'. Later when asked by the worker whether he has been having any sexual problems, he replies 'All my life' and elaborates thus: 'Naturally. You probably suspect, as far as the hair stylist and uh, either one way or another, they're straight or homosexual, something like that...'. Analysis of the full conversation indicates that not only does the patient expect the worker to draw some inference about his sexuality from the mention of the category 'hair stylist', he intends the worker to do so. In this interaction, the patient, who later acknowledges his 'homosexual tendencies', subtly allows the worker an opportunity to pick up on this, but does not explicitly invite the inference. Conversation analysis thus reveals the intricacy and complexity of human communication – in this instance, the ascription of meaning to the social category of 'hair stylist'. It shows how we are able to use categories of social identity as 'resources for social action'. This man uses them to signal something about himself which he may feel is potentially problematic. By giving the subtle clue to the worker, he is able to establish the worker's sensitivity and probable response to the information. If the worker does not notice the clue or reacts unfavourably, the patient can simply move on and not allow any further exploration of this sensitive issue. Clearly, the four maxims do not provide adequate guidance to the participants in this example.

Other attempts to clarify communication have developed process models, which typically distinguish a number of features in order to further analyse them. Probably the most well known is Berlo's (1960) SMCR model, which distinguishes four elements: source (the person who sends), message (the content), channel (the medium of communication) and receiver (the recipient). This model presents a rather static picture of communication and takes little account of feedback from receiver to source. Westley and MacLean (1957) developed a more dynamic model, which allowed for greater responsiveness; however, in both accounts there is relatively little attention given to the influence of social context and culture. Communication theory has focused attention upon the skills required for effective communication but, as Hartley (1993) has noted, 'there is still a common belief that socially skilled action and methods of interpersonal relating are not amenable to training or education. It is still common to hear nurses at all levels say that social skills just come naturally.' This is illustrated by Webb's (1993) account of her own child's admission to hospital, which demonstrates how nurses and doctors often ignore the usual strategies of conversation such as negotiation and bargaining, and use language which disempowers parents. One ward sister, responding to Webb's request to allow her to take her child outside on a hot day, said 'I do allow children from my ward out sometimes'.

The ritualistic conversational styles of the medical profession may be problematic: they may fail to elicit useful information and may sometimes signal a lack of interest in the patient's responses. Chapman (1993) notes a nurse's response to a patient who was perceived as a complainer:

Nurse: Hello, how are you?

Patient: Alright, thank you nurse.

Nurse: That's good (as she moved to the next patient).

If after the general enquiry, the nurse had asked a specific question, such as 'And how is your stomach?', she would have encouraged the patient to respond more specifically and perhaps gained useful information. In this instance, the message to the patient seemed to be 'I am busy and I am not really interested in you'.

The social skills approach to communication developed by Argyle (1983) provides a useful account of the technical aspects of communication and provides a framework for rehearsal and improvement. However, to simply adopt the skills approach to communication would be mistaken. The drawback is that it tends to suggest that all human problems are technical ones, which could be solved by more and better communication. Burgoon, Hunsaker and Dawson (1994) have criticized this tendency: 'People can well understand someone's position and [still] reject the validity of it'; they point out that to focus exclusively upon the quality and extent of communication can detract from the message. Thus, to simply focus upon communication skills alone effectively depoliticizes conflict and disagreement.

NON-VERBAL CODES OF COMMUNICATION

There are a number of other non-verbal codes, which are not languages, but are systematic means of communicating information about meaning, emotion, intent and veracity. It is not the purpose of this book to review these, but their significance should be noted, especially as there is evidence that indicates that these elements convey as much, if not more, of the meaning of utterances than do the actual words themselves (Argyle, 1983). Some of these codes may seem very simple or restricted but they remain important elements in communication. **Kinesics** refers to the study of face and body movement and their meanings. **Paralinguistics** refers to the study of the things which surround or accompany speech but are not actually part of it. These may be hesitations, sighs, silences, grunts and the whole gamut of 'ums' and 'ahs' which are used in conjunction with oral language. **Proxemics** refers to the study of contact, space and the positioning of people and objects within it. It is well established that there is enormous cultural variation in each of these fields, and that they may be a critical element in transcultural communication (Gudykunst and Kim, 1992, Samovar and Porter, 1985). For example, Sue and Sue (1990) have suggested, with regard to different notions of what constitutes appropriate and comfortable space, that a client:

may cause the counsellor to back away because of the closeness taken. The client may interpret the counsellor's behaviour as indicative of aloofness, coldness, or a desire not to communicate...it may even be perceived as a sign of haughtiness and superiority. On the other hand, the counsellor may misinterpret the client's behaviour as an attempt to become inappropriately intimate, a sign of pushiness or aggressiveness.

Sue and Sue, 1990

What is required is a recognition that the use of movement, space, gesture, expression and so on are all culturally conditioned forms of behaviour, which may confirm, contradict or send different messages to those expressed in the verbal language. Interestingly, reports from Argyle (1975) and Pederson (1985) suggest that not only is non-verbal communication harder to control or suppress, but it is perceived as being more reliable than words. Therefore, health and welfare professionals who have not come to terms with issues of sexuality, racial prejudice, disability and so on are unlikely to be able to disguise their perceptions from their clients. In many circumstances, congruency is most likely to be achieved by those workers who are drawn from similar backgrounds to the clients, and who are aware of and have tackled their own prejudices.

CONCLUSION

The primary purpose of this chapter has been to draw attention to the socially constructed nature of language use. By this, I mean the ways in which the meaning of language and the ways in which it is used are derived from tacit understandings and 'rules' that structure ordinary conversation. Much of the work on language in communication has been part of broader studies of human interaction; it has focused upon non-verbal aspects of communication – the presentation of self, the use of space or the presentation and control of information. The need to act upon the information and analysis from the empirical studies of language use is becoming more widely acknowledged, and there is little doubt that training in communication strategies and skills improves performance (Burgoon, Hunsaker and Dawson, 1994). Unfortunately, most of this knowledge is situated at the micro level of social analysis and rarely offers any explicit account of power or pursues the question of cultural difference.

However, the tacit 'rules' and understandings that structure and make sense of our communication are not static. They do not exist outside our minds, but are part of a dynamic social process which operates continuously and is, therefore, continuously open to the possibility of manipulation, misunderstanding and alteration. Conversation analysis has 'shown that ordinary language use is the site for social action: through their talk, people perform such actions as questions, answers, complaints, justifications, mitigations, invitations, acceptances or refusals and so on. They perform a myriad range of social actions' (Widdicombe and Wooffitt, 1995). Nevertheless, we need to go beyond locating these issues solely at the level of the person, since there are other factors which influence both our understanding and our actions in all communication. The most significant of these is power. As we shall see in Chapter 5, the capacity to construct meaning and to shape language use has potentially far-reaching consequences, since it can shape the very concepts that we think with, the ideas that we hold and the behaviour that results.

<table>
<tr><td>5</td><td><h1>Language and power</h1></td></tr>
</table>

Men [*sic*] make their own history but they do not make it just as they please: they do not make it under circumstances chosen by themselves, but under circumstances directly encountered, given and transmitted from the past.

Marx, 1969

To be a 21st century black is not to let the past chain you down. It is to see the future and rewrite it before it even starts.

George, 1994

INTRODUCTION

While these writers differ in their view of the degree of freedom that people have, both emphasize the role of the past in shaping the future and both have recognized how important it is to develop a conscious awareness of this history. Though Marx was writing as a political theorist in the 19th century and George is writing as a black man in 20th-century USA, each points up the significance of ideas and beliefs as crucial elements in asserting power. As we shall see in this chapter, language is the crucial mediator in communicating and constructing our ideas about society.

Unfortunately, within linguistics the question of the relationship of language and power is often focused solely at the interpersonal level of communication. The general tendency has been to examine the ways in which conversational styles reveal differences of power (Ng and Bradac, 1993). Williams (1992), in his sociological critique of linguistic theory, suggests that the issue of power has either been:

- ignored;
- presumed by implicit consensual models of society; or
- subsumed within inadequate structural functionalist theories of society.

For example, he notes that, in cases where one language is replaced by another, the process of change is often characterized by linguists as arising from the actions of formal institutions such as schools and government agencies, but rarely are the bases of these actions explained or challenged. Williams (1992) argues that these formal institutions are presented as 'neutral, abstract' agencies divorced from any political context; 'rather we are presented with an image of consenting individuals bowing to a superior status'.

Many linguists have implicitly or explicitly adopted the types of functionalist approach that tend to describe the events wrought by power, rather than analyse the processes and bases of power itself. Where power is explicitly considered, it is often presented in lopsided ways, with language either totally subsumed by the power of some dominant group such as men (Spender, 1980), or treated asif individuals were free to use language in whatever ways they wished.In this latter view, conversation and meaning are presented as neutral objects, power is simply regarded as a property that individuals possess (Gal, 1979).

The concluding remarks in Chapter 1, on the question of linguistic determinism, that is, the extent to which language precedes thought or thought precedes language, suggested that making this issue an either/or question was not a useful way to proceed. Linguistic determinism is one aspect of the wider debate about the extent to which individuals are determined by external factors or have the capacity of free will. Although Marx was writing about social action, not language, the quotation reveals his appreciation of how we may be acted upon and yet still have the possibility to influence events. I suggest that a similar dialectical approach is required to develop our understanding of the relationship of language to power. Yes, we are presented with patterns of language and meaning that predate our existence, and yes, the actions of others may shape our thoughts and language; but we do not have to accept these patterns and representations. As the quotation from George suggests, all people are shaped by the past but they have some capacity to alter the future. We may become aware of how the language that structures and encapsulates our thought is formed and thus seek to change it.

This chapter explores theoretical and empirical knowledge about the relationship between language and power, from the level of personal communication to the sweep of grand theory. It does not attempt to establish a general theory of power, nor simply incorporate or assume the premises of Marx's political theory, but it does utilize some of his influential analytical devices, namely the dialectic and his development of the concept of ideology (McLellan, 1995).

DEFINING POWER

At its simplest, power can mean the ability of people to further their own interests or aims, to do or get done the things they want. As Ng and Bradac (1993)
note 'It is the kind of concept that most people think they understand intuitively
– until someone asks them to define it'. Ng and Bradac follow a conventional
line in distinguishing between **power to**, meaning the achievement of desired
aims; and **power over**, meaning the ability to make other people act according
to one's aims, that is, to influence, compel or coerce others. In my view,
however, these are not two different types of power. The latter may be seen as a
subdivision of the first, more general statement. Their distinction marks the
difference between those aims that require power over other people and those
that do not, but there are very few instances where the action of one person does
not directly or indirectly affect other people. A doctor's decision to prescribe
one drug rather than another may seem purely a matter of individual discretion
within the prescribing policies of a given health authority, but even within this
framework the exercise of this choice has implications for other patients,
doctors and drug manufacturers.

Power is always relational. That is, it cannot be defined without relating it to
other people or groups who either have it or are subject to its exercise.
Sociologists have distinguished between coercive and consensual forms of
power and some, like Weber (Freund, 1968), have seen authority as the most
significant aspect of social order. Even Marx, who believed that the ruling
classes would always ultimately resort to the most coercive forms of power,
sanctioned in the use of the police or the army, accepted that industrial societies
were not ruled simply by the threat of force: he saw that there was some acceptance on the part of the subject classes of the right of others to rule.

For Marx and his followers, this acceptance was of course manufactured, a
form of false consciousness in which the subject classes were unable to recognize where their true interests lay. In part this false consciousness consisted of
ideologies that legitimized existing social arrangements and thus explained the
apparent contradiction of the poorest class's acceptance and support of those
who exploited and oppressed them. Marx argued that the ruling ideas in capital-
ist society were those of the ruling class, but he never clearly explained how the
false consciousness that supposedly prevents workers from realizing the extent
of their economic exploitation is established.

This idea of manufactured agreement was later developed by Gramsci (1971)
in his theory of **hegemony**, which provided a more sophisticated account of
how ideas were manipulated and structured. Gramsci argued that the powerful
classes maintained their power through the inculcation of their ideas and beliefs
throughout every aspect of social life – 'in other words, the world view of the
ruling class was so thoroughly diffused by its intellectuals as to become the
"common sense" of the whole of society' (McLellan, 1995). Thus, ideologies of
work, law, the family and so on subtly operate to legitimate existing

arrangements. The consequence of the successful spread and incorporation of these hegemonic ideas throughout society is that workers for the most part accept their position because they accept the political and moral values of the ruling class. However, Gramsci did not think that the ruling classes could always impose entirely false ideas, nor did he think their power was absolute. He thought that the powerful classes had to make concessions, because they themselves were sometimes divided and because of the force of working-class demands. Mishra (1977), for example, views the National Health Service as a concession made to the working class in the political turmoil and aftermath of the Second World War.

Many political theorists emphasize ideology as a critical component of power, because of the way in which ideologies construct some patterns of thought and restrict or deny others. Ideologies thus have a legitimating function. That is, they promote certain ideas about how society is organized and thus underpin existing social arrangements. For example, we may believe in the rule of law and the ideology of impartial justice, despite the fact that the definition of offences, the decision to prosecute and the sentences delivered by courts may all be subject to social bias. A detailed account of the considerable development of the concept of ideology undertaken by later theorists like Althusser (1971), Goldman (1964) and Poulantzas (1978) is beyond the scope of this book. Readers who wish to further explore this aspect with regard to welfare services are directed to the work of George and Wilding (1976), Wilding (1982) and Manning (1985). When ideologies are conceptualized as false or inaccurate ideas, the role of language is usually viewed simply as a carrier of meaning (McLellan, 1995), the primary focus being upon how language directly carries and represents power.

However, there is another approach to ideology, which develops the idea of the symbolic role of words and language as representations of people, objects and actions. In these semantic approaches to power, the emphasis is not so much upon the extent to which language conveys ideas about the world that are demonstrably false, but upon the ways in which language itself represents particular meanings. From this perspective, the words we use do not represent one unchanging objective reality but rather construct particular ideas or subjective realities (Hodge and Kress, 1993). This is most clearly appreciated in the processes of identification and naming of things. As we saw in the discussion of categorization in Chapter 2, acts of definition may present a view of the world as appearing to be naturally divided into dual categories such as man/woman, heterosexual/homosexual, and so on. The crucial question is, what is the role of language in creating these ideologies or subjective realities about people and society?

In general, power is better understood as a relative social process than as some absolute or fixed quality (Lukes, 1974, 1986). At the interpersonal level, the ability of senior colleagues to intimidate junior ones is not simply an attribute that they possess as a consequence of their formal occupational role. If they choose to intimidate some people rather than others, it is a social process. The victims may be all those who are formally defined as subordinate, but they may also be selected according to the aggressor's perception of their attractiveness, their likely resistance and so on. The actual incidence of harassment or bullying may also rest upon the weaker person's acceptance or assumption of other constraints upon their own responses. The recognition of this social process should not be seen as an attempt to blame the victim, but is to understand that the fact that power is relational, that it is not the same fixed quality in every situation. Hugman (1991) captures this aspect well: 'It may be anticipated that a white male senior nurse exercises power very differently from a black female nursing assistant, and that both will have a different basis for their actions towards a middle-class white male patient and towards a working-class black female patient.'

As Giddens (1976, 1984) has suggested, there is a reciprocal aspect to all power relations, while some people clearly have more power and resources than others. There is, as Davis (1991) suggests 'some degree of autonomy and dependence in both directions. Power is never a simple matter of "haves and have nots".'

This may seem to be an overstatement, especially when we consider situations such as those involving physical force, where the victim apparently has no option or choice. Nevertheless, we should be careful of overstating power and especially careful of thinking of the 'victims' as completely determined by the actions of more powerful people. We may recognize situations where intimidation continues because the victim decides not to leave their job, report the abuse or retaliate verbally or physically. Powerlessness may arise from the actual imbalance of physical or mental capacity to do any or all these things, but it may also come from some degree of acceptance or unwitting acquiescence in the situation. Davis summarizes this point: 'Compliance is often the result of a decidedly rational assessment of the situation and the viable alternatives; it does not automatically entail agreement'.

It is possible that the same bullying behaviour might be rather less effective when practised upon another subordinate, not because their formal position is any different but because they possess other resources, which allow them to resist or be more resilient in similar circumstances. Research into the accounts offered by children and adults who abuse children (Wolf, 1994) shows that they often spend a considerable amount of time deciding who to abuse and in assessing their relative strength/weakness. It is significant that most efforts at empowerment involve rethinking ideas about what is normal and acceptable behaviour by others and oneself. Power is a social process which is frequently mediated through language; thus the point at which 'the worm turns' is typically when the victim has 'had enough' or has redefined her/his situation as harassment, intimidation or oppression.

There are many resources that can be used to exercise power, as the example of workplace intimidation indicates; 'anything that gives one person or group a degree of control over what others want or need can be a power resource' (Mann, 1983). Charisma, status, formal position, knowledge, ideology, skills and appearance can all operate as power resources; language is unique in being both the transmitter of many of these resources and a resource in its own right. But all resources are relational because their effectiveness depends upon the situations in which their use is attempted.

The next five sections review the most prominent ideas about language and power. In each case the material could arguably have been structured differently, but the organizing principle is a movement from ideas that operate primarily at the individual/interpersonal level to more general theories of power and language. The first three sections are loosely based upon Ng and Bradac's (1993) model of language/power relationship, and draw extensively upon their summaries, while the last two sections are additional models and do not follow their typology. The distinction between creating influence and sustaining power is simply a heuristic means of presenting and understanding the material. For if it is accepted that power is not a static property, then, even when its potential is apparent, the exercise of it can also be seen as a creation.

CREATING INFLUENCE

The research that supports this type of linkage of power and language is predominantly concerned with identifying the features of speech that make a speaker's utterances persuasive or influential. It is the witting and unwitting use of such linguistic features in speech that can be said to create power in situations where no other resource appears to explain the recipients' compliance. The use of argument, logic, reasoning, threats and promises are all obvious devices for getting one's way but there are several less obvious factors that can affect the success of such devices. Each of the following factors has potential significance, but their overall effectiveness depends upon there being no marked incongruence between them in use.

Speech rate

Faster speech rates are generally perceived more favourably than slower ones (Brown, 1980; Miller *et al.*, 1976). Thus slow speakers are thought to be less competent (Street and Brady, 1982) unless the topic is especially technical, and the listeners are not expert, when they are likely to be more favourably disposed to slower rates (Brown, Giles and Thackerar, 1985). Slow speech rates are typically seen as an indication of uncertainty and lack of knowledge or understanding. Interestingly, people whose own speech rates are high are more likely to rate slower speakers unfavourably (Street, Brady and Putman, 1983). As speech rate increases the perception of competence levels off, but surprisingly does not diminish significantly. Though, of course, excessively rapid rates without any other congruent features of expertise are rated negatively. It is probable that perceptions of speech rate when allied to stereotypes of people may combine to reinforce positive or negative attributions; thus, older people who may have slower speech may be perceived as dull and incompetent, whereas college lecturers who speak quickly may be assumed to be intelligent and knowledgeable. The perception of competence in such circumstances is not a one-way process. If a student perceives the rapid speech of a lecturer as evidence of competence, then they may also view their own slowness and hesitation in making notes, or in response to questions from the lecturer, as evidence of their own incompetence.

Language intensity

Intensifiers, that is, words that strengthen messages, can enhance the power of the speaker who uses them. The effectiveness of intensifiers is highly dependent upon other factors. Using emotive words like 'hate', 'despise', 'love', 'adore' and strengtheners like 'new', 'great', 'increased', 'very', 'definitely' does not automatically impress recipients favourably. Their judgement of the speaker's use of such words seems to be strongly linked to more general impressions of the speaker's competence. When the speaker is thought to be competent, then the intensifiers complement that view, but when their competence is in doubt or the expressed attitudes conflict with those of the recipients, then naturally, the use of intensifiers is counterproductive (Miller and Basehart, 1969; Mehrley and McCroskey, 1970; McEwen and Greenburg, 1970). Perhaps the most significant factor is gender. Two different studies have shown that the use of intensifiers is more productive for men than for women (Burgoon, Jones and Stewart, 1975; Burgoon, Birk and Hall, 1991). Ng and Bradac comment that 'There appears to be something about the male role that "allows" men to use strong words and phrases: on the other hand, the female role apparently favours neutral or even weak expressive forms' (Ng and Bradac, 1993). This point about the expectations and attributions made between language and gender is explored later in this chapter.

Communication accommodation: divergence and convergence

As noted in the previous chapter, linguistic accommodation may take two forms, convergence and divergence. Convergence occurs when conversationalists alter their language towards each other's styles. It usually indicates politeness, common purpose, friendliness, empathy and solidarity. Less marked convergence can be observed when people modify their accents towards each other's. This typically is a sign of friendliness, but where there is an imbalance of power the deferential shift towards the language of the dominant person should not be mistaken for convergence, since it is not marked by a **mutual** accommodation. Convergence strengthens persuasive influence between speakers, because it signals similarity, and the conscious use of convergence may enhance this effect (Edwards, 1986; Giles *et al.*, 1977). However, the adoption of lower prestige forms of speech by a person in a position of authority may be perceived by the recipient as patronizing. The defining marker of convergence is that it is usually a mutual adaptation by both speakers.

While divergence may reveal pre-existing power relations between people, it can also create as well as sustain power through its exercise. The conscious use of divergence as an assertion of **otherness** can be a powerful weapon. It may create confusion and disarray and allows at least a temporary advantage to its user, especially when it upsets or challenges the world view of the naïve participant. The classic example frequently cited within linguistics, is the instance of the black doctor stopped by a white policeman in the USA. During the course of the questioning, the police officer, to the surprise of the doctor, deliberately refuses to acknowledge his professional title and status by persistently addressing him as 'boy'. The officer uses this language not simply to assert his formal role but also to derogate by racist language the doctor's status as a person (Ervin-Tripp, 1972). This divergent use of language creates a powerful advantage for the officer and, through the devaluation of the black man, sustains racism. The effects of divergence are greatest when the recipient is unaware of the potential difference about to be displayed.

When the potential recipient is aware of the possibility of a 'put down', its effectiveness is greatly diminished. The experience of discrimination by many ethnic minorities leads them as individuals to be wary of such encounters. This heightened awareness of the actions of more powerful people is a common feature of oppression. (It can even be seen in the behaviour of abused children who sometimes display a 'frozen watchfulness' in the presence of their abuser and other adults.)

REVEALING AND SUSTAINING POWER

When a person speaks, we are usually able to immediately identify certain things about her/him; geographical origins, social class, gender, and even in some instances age and occupation. The experience of a friend who recently gained promotion illustrates this. Prior to his first management meeting his immediate superior advised him to keep quiet, with the words, 'they might wonder whether you know what you are doing, but they will not know for sure unless you open your mouth'. This might simply be seen as the cautious advice of an experienced old-hand to a rookie, but for the fact, that my friend spoke with an obvious rural accent whereas virtually all his new colleagues spoke English with the higher status accent of Received Pronunciation. Thus, when we listen and when we speak, language reveals information about other people and ourselves. This language may reveal information about how powerful/powerless we are in relation to other people in the conversation.

Language and gender

The quotation from Ng and Bradac included in the 'Language intensity' subsection suggested that the gender roles of men and women led to different expectations and evaluations of their speech. However this aspect of language and power needs to be considered carefully. As was noted in Chapter 2, the evidence on speech patterns is not universally accepted as demonstrating that all men and all women do in fact speak differently. Cameron (1992) has typified the supposedly typical features of women's speech as disfluency, unfinished sentences, illogical construction of speech, questions rather than statements, cooperative strategies rather than competitive ones and a tendency to speak less than men in mixed groups. Lakoff (1975) has argued that women have been socialized into subordinate roles and that they are taught language and types of speech pattern which do not challenge or confront male dominance. Instead, both reflect and reinforce their oppression. In a similar vein, Fishman (1978) has argued that there is a normative component to women's use of language, in that, as Williams (1992) states, 'Being a woman in the conventional sense is incompatible with asserting control'.

The evidence which suggests that women interrupt other speakers less, use more tag questions, such as 'isn't it?' and hesitate more is frequently derived from small, unrepresentative studies. These have sometimes ignored other important variables such as formal role and education (Cameron, 1992; Ng and Bradac, 1993). Cameron claims that such variations, to the extent that they exist, are misunderstood and misinterpreted; she notes that disfluency, hesitation and unfinished sentences are common in the speech of both women and men. Cameron argues that the supposed illogicality of women's speech arises from androcentric (male-centred) definitions of reasoning, and that much of the variation cited in support of women's language is more accurately viewed as being indicative of low power and status. Thus, these features may be heard in the speech of powerless men too. Her point is that these variations are not primarily evidence of gender difference *per se*, but evidence of powerlessness. Thus women, who as a group are generally less powerful, exhibit these variations more frequently and the variations should be understood as evidence of gender subordination, not innate sexual difference. Interestingly, some feminists also contend that women characteristically speak differently, and prefer their supposedly less assertive and cooperative style to that used by men. Consequently, they have tried to develop this preferred style. Arguably, they are engaged in a revaluation of the negative attribution as positive. The implications of such strategies in the creation of positive self-identity were noted in Chapter 3. There is, however, a more significant point with regard to the expectations that we may have, and the attributions that we make: it may not be a matter of irrefutable fact that men and women speak differently, but it is beyond doubt that many people expect and believe that they do (Mulac and Lundell, 1986; Mulac, Lundell and Bradac, 1986; Tannen, 1986).

While the older negative attributions made to women's speech – often described as shrill in tone, trivial in content and frivolous in thought – are rarely heard today (Coates, 1993; Cameron, 1992); unfavourable comparisons with the supposed coherence and gravitas of men's language are still made. It is well known that Margaret Thatcher, in her attempts to appear more authoritative and powerful, deliberately lowered the pitch of her voice. There is also evidence that the written and spoken language produced by men is perceived as being more dynamic, while that produced by women is thought to be more aesthetic (Mulac, 1976; Mulac and Lundell, 1982, 1986).

Language, perception of position and expectancy

Within communications theory, the uncertainty reduction thesis of Berger and Calabrese (1975) hypothesizes that a prime element in all communication is the desire to reduce uncertainty and increase predictability. Ng and Bradac suggest that the extent to which speakers will tend to do this depends upon their perceptions of each other's power. If the other person is more powerful, then the consequences of misunderstanding could be more problematic. Thus one might suppose, the speech of the person who shoulders the burden of clarification reveals the imbalance of power. This seems an apt description of many interactions between professionals and clients, where there is an imbalance of power. Yet clients typically ask fewer rather than more questions. It may be that uncertainty is to some degree constrained by the expectations of the situation; therefore strategies to reduce it are not required. Alternatively, the power imbalance may be so great as to effectively silence the powerless client, who wishes to receive the professional's service and realizes that further questioning may be counterproductive. A working-class patient's perception of her/himself as a burden may be evidenced by a reluctance to 'bother the doctor', whereas the more assertive language of a middle-class patient indicates a perception of equality, and thus expects, if not demands, the attention of the doctor.

The expectations that people bring to their communications go further than just the perception of power, to expectations of the actual language that is likely to be used in particular circumstances. Power is associated with expectations of vocabulary, syntax, pronunciation and so on. Ng and Bradac suggest that powerful people are expected to use powerful (i.e. high-prestige) language and the opposite applies to powerless people. Verbal performance that is consistent with these expectations reinforces them, while performance that contradicts them alters perceptions of competence. Such expectations need not always be previously established; the opening speaker in a conversation may set the style, which shapes the expectations of subsequent speakers. If they do not adopt the expectation, they may be perceived both by the first speaker and by any other participants as being less competent and thus less persuasive or powerful.

Casting and roles

Siegal (1990) has noted that, when children are in Piagetian-type clinical interviews with authority figures whom they assume to be powerful and knowledgeable, they expect of the questions to be relevant and thus attempt to answer accordingly – consequently, they will change their answers from one question to another. Because of their desire to conform, they will not be consistent in their answers even when they should be. This type of response is frequently seen in the behaviour of young schoolchildren who, in their desire to please their teacher, will spontaneously put their hands up to answer a question and then sometimes provide a totally irrelevant answer. Such socialized role expectations also have powerful effects upon adult interactions.

CONCEALING POWER

The euphemistic use of language to obscure issues or avoid direct acknowledgement of the fact that power is being used is a common device for avoiding confrontation. Misrepresentation or watering down of information can effectively depoliticize sensitive issues about which there is, or may be, considerable conflict. Ironically, instead of acknowledging that it is their own interests which are being served, the justification often given by those who adopt such strategies is that they are considering someone else's feelings or interests. These patronizing presumptions are probably most common when the direct acknowledgement of selfish motives is deemed unacceptable, as in the helping professions. Among the excuses that I have heard given by some professionals for resisting the presence of parents at child protection conferences was that the parents would not understand the proceedings and 'anyway it would be too upsetting for them'.

Mitigating devices

These are the mildest forms of concealment, in that they are attempts to ameliorate the potentially negative consequences of exercising power or communicating information. Fraser (1980) defines mitigation as attempts 'to soften the effects of an order, ease the blow of bad news, make a criticism more palatable...'. Ng and Bradac (1993), building upon the work of Fraser (1980) and Holmes (1984), have suggested that all mitigation strategies can be subsumed under two headings, **indirectness** and **tentativeness**.

Indirectness

Indirectness is part of the repertoire of communication competence that speakers learn from childhood, and there is considerable cultural variation from one language to another. It is primarily a device for depersonalizing communication, so that criticisms, requests and statements are apparently distanced from the immediate context of the conversationalists. Indirectness serves to maintain the listener's sense of independence and autonomy. Typically, interrogative questions about someone's performance are phrased in a task-centred manner. For example, a manager in a residential setting may ask a subordinate whether the beds have been made, either **directly**, as in 'Have you made the beds?', or **indirectly**, as in 'Have the beds been made?' The worker may respond directly, 'No, I haven't done them yet,' or indirectly, 'No, they haven't.' If there are only two people present, there is little doubt in the worker's mind that the indirect question is in fact a direct request or reminder, but if the worker decides to respond directly and wishes to maintain appropriate deference, then the addition of a hedge word like 'yet' avoids offending the manager. Otherwise the minimalist response 'No, I haven't done them,' may be construed as being too assertive and challenging. Obviously there will be other cues, such as the tone of voice and the general demeanour of the participants, which will also provide important information as to how they may construe each other's intentions and meanings.

Understanding the meaning of indirect communication requires a shared appreciation of such routinized devices. In the above example, the question may also be understood as a direct request. Other routinized forms of indirectness can be seen when direct declarations such as 'I am hungry' are meant and understood as requests, i.e. 'Feed me'. People who learn English as a second language may not always appreciate, or have learned, the significance of these indirect devices, so there is considerable potential for misunderstanding.

Similarly, people from other linguistic cultures may perceive first-language English speakers to be rude and insensitive, because they are accustomed to a greater degree of indirectness. For example, the direct refusal or denial of a request made between colleagues, friends or business associates may be perceived as hostile and impolite, especially when the negative response is construed as leading to a loss of face or dignity. The frustrations of British businessmen in their dealings with Japanese companies, whom they perceive to be excessively cautious, indirect and less than frank, have been a rich source of misunderstanding. It is worth noting that, from a European perspective, the stereotypical perception of the English as being the nation of 'perfidious Albion' may derive from differing conventions of directness, especially in regard to the expression of disagreement.

Our understanding of the repertoire and function of indirect devices begins very early in our lives. Young children learn that they are not expected to tell adults what to do. They learn that indirectness is the preferred style of communicating their desires, perhaps by thinly masking them as requests for favours; switching from directives to questions, such as 'Can I have some chocolate?' instead of 'Buy me some sweets'. Ervin-Tripp and Gordon (1986) suggest that this aspect of indirectness is usually accomplished by the age of 4 years. Many indirect devices, such as irony and understatement, are routinized and learned generally, but some are more specific, being confined to smaller groups of people, perhaps as a means of signalling in-group status.

This issue of shared understandings and perceptions, that is, of shared context, discussed in Chapter 3, is a critical element in communication. Smaller speech communities generally have higher levels of implicit understanding, and hence many items in conversation may be left unsaid, or are inferred from the context. The mutual knowledge that underpins the communication allows speakers to judge the meaning of other people's language. For example, an implicit threat or promise is not just recognized but is also assessed as to its probability. This in turn depends upon the listener's perception of the power of the other person to action the meaning.

Indirectness can be deliberately used to disrupt communication and to deny information. Politicians frequently avoid answering questions they feel compromise or commit them, by being indirect in their responses. Typically, a specific question is answered with a generality. Social workers too, are not immune from this: one worker, after leaving a child protection case conference, in response to the question 'How did it go?', replied 'Oh, everyone turned up.' The question, however, was intended to elucidate what decision had been made about the child.

Tentativeness

Mitigating devices which employ tentativeness can be used with both direct and indirect language. Variations in the intonation and stress put upon words can be used to mitigate the effects upon the listener. Falling and rising intonations within utterances are one way of conveying tentativeness. The bluntness of a directive may be mitigated by using a wheedling form of rising intonation which changes the meaning, to something closer to a request – for example, 'Pass me the pillow'. Directives that order other people to do things are often mitigated by using a gentle tone which suggests consideration and tact. Kramarae (1982) and Brazil, Coulthard and Johns (1980), have noted how, among English speakers, higher vocal pitches and rising intonations may suggest deference, through an association with the speech patterns of children, and girls in particular.

Another common form of tentativeness is the use of reservations, which mitigate the force of statements by the use of such devices as **tag questions**, **disclaimers** and **qualifiers**. Tag questions like 'Isn't it?', 'Don't you agree?' and 'You won't mind if I go first, will you?' typically take the form of riders added on to the end of statements. In such cases, a degree of compliance has already been presumed by the speaker. Disclaimers, which often precede utterances, such as 'I'm not sure, but...' and 'I missed the last meeting, but my understanding was...', appear to indicate reservations by the speaker about the status of her/his utterances, but the intention is to query the anticipated course of action. This, of course, is one of the most common devices for disrupting the progress of formal meetings.

Qualifiers are devices for expressing uncertainty about the accuracy or truth of propositions and are usually signalled by the use of parenthetical verbs like 'I gather' or 'I suppose'. They can also take the form of hedges in words and phrases, like 'allegedly', 'sort of', 'a bit like' and 'sometimes might'. In each instance, the speaker is avoiding full responsibility for the validity of the proposition contained in her/his utterance.

Traditionally, mitigating devices of indirectness and hesitation are presumed to be evidence of powerlessness (O'Barr and Atkins, 1980; Cameron, 1992) but, as Ng and Bradac (1993) have shown, they can also be used as ways of concealing power. Perhaps it would be wise to consider their use by relatively powerful individuals as linguistic wolves in sheep's clothing. However, it is probable that, in such circumstances, the efficacy of mitigation depends not so much upon the apparent disguise of power as on the realization that its crude exercise may be counterproductive. Both Marx and Gramsci noted that the appearance or illusion of consent provided a stronger base for exploitation than crude coercion.

Finally, it is worth considering what motives underlie the use of mitigating devices. Ng and Bradac suggest that there are two types of primary motive. The first type is self-serving, which occurs when mitigation is used to promote personal aims. These may occur when a worker has power and intends to use it, but does not wish to unnecessarily antagonize the service user. The second type is altruistic, and is used primarily to promote or protect the feelings of the recipient. Ng and Bradac accept that a mitigation utterance might serve both motives, but maintain that normally one motive is dominant. For example, a psychiatrist might say to a potentially suicidal patient 'I'm afraid that I think you are a danger to yourself', in a manner and tone of voice that is gentle and caring. The patient's thoughts and feelings are being addressed, but the primary aim may be to convey the fact that compulsory detention is being considered.

Misrepresentation and masking devices

Hugman (1991), in stating that 'the language of professionalism frequently serves to obscure the issue of power', echoes the scepticism of George Bernard Shaw, who described the professions as a conspiracy against the common people. This negative perception of professional power is widely held, yet is infrequently acknowledged by human service professionals unless it is clothed in the garb of normalization, empowerment or radical theory. As we shall see in the final chapter, it is imperative to raise our own awareness of how language may mask the meanings of our actions.

Human service professionals may have good cause to be uncertain and uneasy about coping with violence and aggression in their workplace. Yet, for example, to describe the rapid tranquillization of aggressive psychiatric patients as 'treatment' (Pilowsky, 1994) is to obscure the meaning of the action, which is primarily about control rather than therapy.

Though masking devices are typically viewed as the preserve of those with power, they may be used by those who are relatively powerless, in order to reduce their vulnerability to the actions of their superiors. In both instances, the devices confer power by representing the world and events within it in ways that are congruent with the ambitions and intentions of the person using them, thus depoliticizing the exercise of power and obscuring the fact of its use. Depoliticization is commonly achieved by depersonalizing the actions or intentions of those who exercise power. Often, the welfare of the patient or the greater good of the organization becomes the expressed rationale for certain actions, rather than a more explicit identification of personal gain.

Misrepresentation

Obviously, lies and falsehoods are explicit forms of masking in that they consciously seek to deny the truth of a situation. Ng and Bradac suggest that lies are usually only required when concealment is impossible. However, listeners may be misled by other devices that misrepresent the speaker's views and perceptions. Perhaps one of the most common forms of misrepresentation is the omission of pertinent information from communication.

Sometimes the speaker may communicate her/his intentions or perceptions but distort them by exaggeration, minimization or equivocation, so that the listener misunderstands the extent of speaker's involvement in events or misreads the strength of the speaker's position. Clearly, if either of these reactions is induced, then potential reaction, opposition and conflict are minimized. Devious messages may 'exploit the slippage that exists between the pragmatic and semantic dimensions' (Ng and Bradac, 1993) of language, that is, between the nominal and the actual meanings of words and sentences. Thus, in response to a question, the respondent may deliberately misconstrue the meaning, so that the answer appears truthful yet does not reveal the desired information.

Masking

The use of particular words and their associated meanings, as well as their position in the sentence structure, can also be effectively used for masking. The descriptions and analysis of these forms of masking derive largely from the work of Fowler *et al.* (1979), Hodge and Kress (1993), Halliday (1976) and Habermas (1979). These writers attempted to unearth the processes of communication by means of close textual analysis of language, its rules of presentation and its associated structures of meaning. From such analyses they interpret the implicit ideas and views of reality carried by the communication. The import of their work relates to the more general question of which 'realities' we use to understand the world; it is discussed further in the next section. For the moment,

I shall concentrate upon the lower levels of their analyses of masking which Ng and Bradac (1993) summarize thus: 'Masking does not withhold true information or present false information as if true, rather it presents true information in an incomplete or partial way under the cover of one or more literary masks.'

Truncation is one device which masks reality by omitting explicit information and leaving particular items as tacit or implicit in communication. The unspoken bits that are missing are not redundant information but often critical aspects of the communication. Thus the statement 'I know where you live' communicates more than its literal content: it can imply some form of unspecified threat.

Permutation, another masking device, operates by the manipulation of sentence structures to alter the meaning or emphasis conveyed. If, as is common in standard English, the first idea conveyed in a sentence is the dominant one, then switching the position of the idea may affect the listener's perception of the information they receive. This is a common tactic of newspaper headline writers, who manipulate the ordering of ideas in sentences in order to make news. For example, these two sentences assign different prominence to the idea 'social worker':

Social worker fails to protect child from brutal beating by stepfather.
Stepfather's beating kills child on social worker's At Risk list.

Thus, culpability is more definitely assigned to the social worker in the first sentence than in the second.

Generalizations are devices that create the impression of a wider frame of reference, whereas the meaning of the statements refer specifically to particular people, things or events. A doctor's utterance, 'How are we feeling today?', appears to be inclusive, suggesting an identification between the doctor and the patient's state of health. Of course, only the patient is ill, and the doctor may use the collective 'we' simply in order to show sympathy with the patient's condition. It may, however, be a subtle attempt to influence the patient's response, since it implies that the patient is responsible for the doctor's feelings too, and thus the patient is encouraged to reply positively in response to the more powerful person's inquiry. Statements like 'We will all have to make sacrifices from now on' suggest an ulterior motive, since they are typically made by more powerful people to those who are less powerful. Such statements attempt to be inclusive and draw upon the stock of ideas that we have about in-group membership; they attempt to 'induce in the addressee a sense of affiliation and obligation' (Ng and Bradac, 1993). Another form of generalization is to use abstract words to replace more specific ones. Abstract descriptions tend to be harder to contradict and seem to be more enduring. For example, in disciplinary proceedings, the accusation of 'unprofessional conduct' conveys a more negative impression than a specific allegation that 'Nurse X failed to write up the patient's observation records'.

Nominalization is a masking device that typically depersonalizes the exercise of power. This is achieved by changing sentences from ones that identify action through verbs and verb clauses to statements that use a noun or noun phrase. This has the effect of changing statements from ones that indicate that an activity is being carried out by one person upon another to an event that has no named participants. For example: 'The Director of Social Services will discipline social workers who fail to follow the standard procedures' may be replaced with 'Failure to follow procedures is a disciplinary offence'. Nominalization is similar to the indirect device of distancing, since it also tends to depoliticize situations where conflicts of interest or disparities of influence exist. It makes the exercise of power seem like something which is inevitable and immutable, rather than a consequence of someone's actions.

Finally, it should be noted that obscurity and difficulty in comprehending the meanings of others is not invariably a sign of duplicity or misrepresentation. Besides the limited capacity of some people to communicate effectively when they are using a second language, there are a number of congenital and acquired conditions that diminish clarity and directness. Some forms of brain damage and 'mental illness' are also accompanied by problems of communication.

DEFINING THE LANGUAGE

The choice of language is one of the most obvious signs of power. The selection of one type or form of language rather than another, practically and symbolically asserts the dominance of that language user. Thus, choice reveals power and also reinforces it, by excluding or marginalizing those who cannot speak the chosen language or prefer not to. Edwards (1994) cites the case of a French scientist who failed to gain promotion at the Centre National de la Recherche Scientifique because of his lack of publications in English! English is now dominant throughout the scientific community and most scientists recognize this, as an article in one of the most influential journals, *Nature*, entitled 'Publish in English or perish' indicates (Bakewell, 1992).

When governments seek to manipulate the choice of language they frequently marginalize existing language groups, who become linguistic minorities (Bourhis, 1984). Unfortunately, the suppression of particular languages has been a relatively commonplace occurrence. Within Britain, both Welsh and British Sign Language have been treated in this way. From the Act of Union in 1536, Welsh was regarded unfavourably and its use became proscribed in official matters of government and law. By the 19th century, Welsh was primarily the language of unofficial life, that is, the home, chapel and village (Davies, 1994). The 1870 Education Act required English to be spoken in schools and the 'Welsh Not' was used to punish pupils who spoke Welsh. This was similar to the 'Token' used at the same time in France, where pupils caught speaking languages other than French were made to wear a 'token' around their neck;

whoever wore the token at the end of the day was punished by the teacher. Pupils could only escape this fate by telling the teacher of another child speaking the forbidden language and so transferring the token to them (Bourhis, 1984)! Measures like these led to feelings of distrust among Welsh speakers and to shame among Welsh children about their native language (Pugh, 1994b).

The effects upon personal and group identity when languages are suppressed and derogated were reviewed in Chapter 3. The damaging effects of suppression upon attainment are exemplified in the case of British Sign Language (BSL), which was systematically denied to deaf children for nearly 80 years. From 1800–1880 deaf schools and clubs teaching and using BSL flourished but, following the Congress of Milan in 1880, its use was discouraged, and was prohibited in many schools. The cult of oralism and the accompanying view that BSL was not really a language but simply a poor imitation of English had many damaging effects upon deaf people and their linguistic community. In some schools, deaf children's hands were tied behind their backs to prevent them from signing. The success of 19th-century deaf schools in preparing their pupils for employment was severely undermined. 'A hundred years later, a survey ... showed that the average reading age of the deaf school leaver was 8.75 years; the speech of 90% of deaf children was described as unintelligible; and their lip-reading skill was found to be no better than that of hearing children (who had never been taught to use this form of communication)' (Ladd, 1991).

People who continued to use BSL were referred to as the 'stupid deaf' or the 'less intelligent deaf' (Ladd, 1991). The failure to acquire a complete symbolic language of any sort would, as McCrone proposes, result in an inability to be able to think and process thought optimally (Chapter 1). Even in supposedly more enlightened times, BSL users continue to be disadvantaged. The emphasis upon integration in the 1981 Education Act threatens the existence of deaf schools, and the virtual debarring of deaf people from teaching in them undermines the teaching and use of the most effective language for deaf people. In most situations where minority language users are expected to integrate, this is almost invariably a one-way process, where the minority are expected to adapt to the majority, but little or no adaptation is made in the other direction. Chapter 3 explored the implications for individual and group identity when language becomes the significant factor in defining who belongs and who does not in a society, and also outlined some of the ways in which minorities may react to their marginalization.

In Chapter 2 the discussion of attitudes showed how unquestioned assumptions about the normality and superiority of English have led to the demise and decline of other languages in Britain and the USA. In these instances, the devaluation of minority languages was not always a planned consequence of the actions of government. However, there are instances, as in the 19th century, when the rise of nationalism was accompanied with the assertion that a nation should speak with one tongue. The notion of the desirability of a monolingual state is still prevalent. In the 1920s, the modern Turkish state was established, with the imposition of the Turkish language and a new alphabet. More recently, Namibia, a former colony of Germany and South Africa, decided to adopt English as its language, despite the fact that only about 2% of the population spoke it. To select one or another of the different tribal languages would have been divisive, and German and Åfrikaans were disregarded because they were unwanted reminders of former colonial status.

Language shifts reveal changes in political power, and this is best illustrated by the case of Québec province in Canada, where the rise to power of the Parti Québecois led to the declaration of French as the sole official language for the province, where fewer than 17% of the population were first-language English speakers. Though the usual direction of language planning has typically been towards a territorial monolingualism, there are exceptions to this. In South Africa, diversity was encouraged by the former racist government in order to foster disunity among the various ethnic groups. Thus, the various African languages were encouraged rather than suppressed (Trudgill, 1983).

Opportunities to define the language that is spoken occur in more limited situations. For example, jargon is typically used by specialist groups to enhance accuracy in communication, but it also serves to signify their common knowledge or status. Thus, the people using the jargon differentiate themselves from other non-group members. Furthermore, jargon may also serve to distance professionals from their service users, and protect them from the painful realities of their work (Satyamurti, 1979). The opportunity to define the language in which services are provided is frequently unrecognized. Because of the presumption that most people can or will speak English, a conscious decision to provide a monolingual service is rarely made. The result is that relatively few services have any explicit policy on language: it remains a peripheral issue. Whatever the reasons for this, the consequences of restricting or denying access to a service by virtue of language can be extremely harmful.

The Health Education Authority (HEA) survey *Black and Minority Ethnic Groups in England* (1995) found that the health of many Afro-Caribbean, Indian, Pakistani and Bangladeshi communities is being seriously damaged by linguistic and cultural barriers. A similar survey (Smaje, 1995) confirmed that health authorities frequently neglect the needs of minority ethnic groups. The most common problems were lack of knowledge about health education, lack of knowledge about services and subsequent lack of take-up of them. For example, while 85% of all women in the UK have had a cervical smear at some time, only 70% of Indian women, 54% of Pakistani women and 40% of Bangladeshi women have ever been checked. While there are difficulties arising from cultural factors, such as different expectations of the medical service, the predominant problem is one of language. Ethnic minority respondents to the HEA survey typically overestimated their own degree of competence in English. For example: 'While 85% of people of Indian origin, 72% of Pakistani and 59% of Bangladeshi said they could speak English, when it came to the survey 70% of the Bangladeshis, 50% of the Pakistanis and 30% of the Indians had to be interviewed in their mother [*sic*] tongue' (Hall, 1995). Their problems did not end there: many respondents also had difficulty reading, or could not read, English. By reason of language, these people were effectively barred from access to health care and health advice. A smaller survey of social service provision in the borough of Tower Hamlets, in London's East End (Ali, Momen and Bhuia, 1995), found very low user-rates among the area's ethnic minority groups. Despite comprising 37% of the borough's population, they formed only 4.5% of the service users. For example, Bangladeshis formed 23% of the local population, yet comprised only 1% of those receiving community care. Thus, important services in day and residential care, occupational therapy and domiciliary provision were underused by them.

DEFINING THE DISCOURSE

Defining the discourse or, more accurately, defining the nature of the discourse refers to the ways in which language can be used to shape the sets of meanings used to think, understand and communicate with. The term **discourse** has many meanings and in its narrowest sense refers only to stretches of narrative in communication. However, following the work of the French writers Foucault (1967, 1972) and Derrida (1987), the phrase **discourse analysis** has come to mean an examination not of the literal meanings of words in communication but of the broader ideas and representations of the world that are carried by passages of words and text. The power of discourse derives from the way in which consciousness itself is structured, usually without any awareness that the things which can be said and thought, are in some sense, constrained. This aspect is captured in the following sentences:

> The structure of speech, writing and action influences what can be said, written and done. In other words, there is a framework in social life, so familiar that we are barely conscious of it, so insistent that we cannot choose to avoid or reject its rules, which makes it possible or impossible to speak about a particular issue or object. This framework is discourse.
>
> *Rojek, Peacock and Collins, 1988*

For example, Thomson and Scott (1991), in their analysis of how young women learn about sex and develop their sexual identity, describe what they term 'the protective discourse', which develops between mothers and their daughters. This discourse is based upon the mother's fears for their daughter's welfare, but passes on negative ideas about sex and sexuality. In 'the absence of more positive information, it serves to support the passive model of female sexuality entrenched in school sex education', thus limiting the daughters' perception of their choices about sex. They are left with a stark choice between simply answering 'yes' or 'no' to the advances of men, who have learnt a different discourse, which presents them with more active and predatory ideas of sexuality. A discourse, therefore, not only carries particular ideas but denies other possibilities. The denial of alternative ideas occurs largely through the omission of these other possibilities, but is also achieved by virtue of the authority of those who iterate and reiterate the discourse. Discourse analysis is as much about what is not said as what is said: it reveals implicit meanings and assumptions about the world that we are not always aware of.

There is a long history of attempts to reveal hidden meanings in words and language, from symbolism to psychoanalysis, but there are obvious problems with approaches that infer meaning in this way. For example, Freud's theory of the development of sexuality has been widely criticized, especially for the concepts of the Electra and Oedipus complexes. Freud thought that these complexes arose from the unsuccessful repression of the developing child's sexual desires. He believed that these desires began with narcissistic self-love, developed through homosexual attraction to one's own sex, then into a hetero-sexual desire for one's (opposite sex) parent, which later became externalized to others. The difficulty, clearly, is that this is a somewhat circular explanation, which is not open to disproof. An individual who admits such past attraction is taken as proof of the theory, while the apparently contradictory denial of another person is explained as the result of having successfully repressed such forbidden urges. Thus, even the exception is hailed as confirmation of the theo-retical rule! Marx's conception of false consciousness is similarly not open to test, since it also forms a closed loop of reasoning.

The proponents of discourse analysis rebut this form of criticism by, first, not claiming to have revealed the 'truth'. They do not assume that there is a single objective reality. They accept that their analysis may be seen simply as one among a multiplicity of possible realities, another perspective upon the situa-tion. Discourse analysis is a theoretical approach which eschews positivistic notions of objectivity and proof: these are seen as social constructions too. Second, discourse analysts would claim some degree of generalization for their interpretations, by demonstrating that specific outcomes arise from particular discourses of meaning. There may be no objective reality, but they do believe that there are more or less useful or effective ways of understanding and repre-senting the world. Thus, they claim some preferential status for their version, since its validity can be attested by the social actions that flow from the preva-lence of particular forms of discourse. Much of the writing of discourse theo-rists is extremely opaque and is open to the very criticism that they have levelled at earlier theorists of power, that of reductionism, where all aspects of social life are reduced to a single dominant variable – power. Giddens (1984) criticizes this tendency to present power as a 'mysterious phenomenon, that hovers everywhere and underlies everything'.

I have used the term 'discourse' to refer to any use of language which struc-tures the meanings and ideas about the world, usually in ways that are not liter-ally expressed in the text, but are implicit. Discourse refers to both passages of communication and the meanings that are conveyed or denied by them, and also to the shared understandings that we use to make sense of the utterances of other people. The example in Chapter 1 of the Asian woman who is unable to understand the psychiatrist's question, 'how are you in yourself?' reveals a specific medical discourse. This discourse conceptualizes mental health as an individual phenomenon, whereas the woman's own discourse reveals an alternative perception of what being healthy means. The major distinguishing factor, other than the content of the discourse, is the relative degree to which each of them is able to impose their version upon the other.

Rojek, et al. (1988) have argued that, 'the language of social workers is not neutral. It is evocative of a historically specific set of professionally received ideas and codes of intervention which organize the professional world.' They suggest, for example, that words like 'respect', 'community' and 'self-determination' are part of the received discourse imparted in professional training. A discourse profoundly influenced by humanism. These potentially powerful words, which are more akin to rhetoric than 'reality', are part of a framework of ideas, which assume the basic similarity of all humans; whereas, there may be many dimensions of difference between them. Furthermore, this received discourse conceives of the professional as being a powerful figure, someone at the centre of the action – saving children, alleviating poverty, dispensing advice and so on. This may bear little resemblance to the actuality of some areas of practice, where interventions may only be marginally effective in changing a person's situation, and ignores the common public perception that social workers, in particular, are people who make things worse, rather than better

This perception of centrality operates in many spheres: Campbell (1994) has suggested that a common feature, shared by both left and right wing critics of 'political correctness', is a perception of themselves as the agents of change not as the subjects for change! They are reluctant to acknowledge that they may be part of the person's problem, rather than the solution (Bor et al., 1993). Furthermore, while their perception of self-importance tends to obscure the patient's point of view, they may fail to grasp that what they think and do is sometimes simply irrelevant.

Within the health professions, resistance to administrative change, to internal markets and so on, is not simply resistance to the loss of professional autonomy, but to a threatening economic discourse. Similarly, when the scientism upon which doctors' professional power is based is threatened by an awareness of the limits of knowledge, it may be preserved by resort to the claim that their professionalism operates in the 'best interests' of the patient. Thus, Electro-Convulsion Therapy (ECT) continues to be used despite no demonstrable scientific explanation of its supposedly beneficial effects.

Simile and metaphor

At a lower level of analysis, similes and metaphors may be seen as devices that shape discourse at the micro level of interaction, that is, the particular words and parts of speech that are employed to shape patterns of meaning. Simile is a device that describes one thing in terms of another. Thus, a calm sea crossing is 'like a millpond', or a passive patient is 'like a baby'. These similes are marked by the word 'like', which signals the supposed similarity with another object or person. Obviously, there are risks in their use. In the latter case, it arises from the infantilization of the adult, but this form of identifying reference is easily recognized. Metaphor is a more powerful figure of speech, in which there is a less obvious identification of one thing with another, such as 'she was an angel' and 'men are animals'. In referring to 'animals', the metaphor relies for its effect upon a common knowledge of which animal characteristics are supposed to be highlighted – in this instance, perhaps, aggressiveness and impulsiveness (Ng and Bradac, 1993).

Metaphors are culturally bound and reflect particular values, for example 'time is money'. Implicit in their use are models of perception; thus the phrase 'things are looking up' not only conveys the message that things are improving but also reflects the idea that 'up' is good. The identification of the colour black with bad things is frequently used metaphorically, in a way which reflects and reinforces the negative connotation given to all people and things black. The power of metaphors derives from the models which they provide for under-standing, thinking and communicating about the world. Sontag (1978, 1988) has described how illness can be viewed as a metaphor about the moral state of a person or society. She describes how the dread meanings attached originally to tuberculosis became linked to cancer and, latterly, AIDS. The plague metaphor invokes ideas of invasion and threat. This has the effect of further stigmatizing already marginalized groups such as homosexual men and black immigrants. In a similar manner, Foucault (1967) has argued that the moral meanings origi-nally attached to leprosy, such as the notion that it was a mark of God's disfavour, were later transferred to madness. The notion of contamination and a belief in the risk of infection were used to justify the exclusion from 'normal' society of those who seemed to pose a threat. In his view, it was no coincidence that the oldest asylums were often built upon the sites of old leprosariums and inherited the symbolic meanings attached to the practice of social isolation and exclusion. Much of the power of metaphor comes from the way in which the meanings that they carry seem natural and thus pass unnoticed and unques-tioned.

Man-made discourse?

Spender (1980), the feminist writer, has persuasively outlined what she thinks the consequence of the unquestioned 'naturalness' of language has been for women, which is that, in a patriarchal world where men have constructed language and its meaning, they have imposed a masculine world-view upon all those who use language. Thus, women are either alienated, in the sense that they have internalized a skewed and inaccurate world-view, or are effectively silenced, since their experiences cannot be adequately represented in this alien language. Women have no alternative but to use the conceptual structures and ideas embedded within the male language. This is the determinism of the Sapir–Whorf hypothesis writ large.

Spender's position has been severely criticized by Black and Coward (1990), who think that the depiction of power and disadvantage portrayed is too simplistic. They note that women are not the only victims in society and that the simple idea of one group (men) having power over another group (women) fails to capture the complexity of a social world in which there are many dimensions of power and many groups who may be disadvantaged by it. They note that some women, by virtue of their class or employment, are in fact able to wield power over men as well as other women. Spender's error in this respect is to elevate a single dimension of power and disadvantage into a rigid, unvarying certainty. This ignores the possibility that the position of any given individual may be determined by other interacting factors such as age, class and disability.

Black and Coward do not doubt that men as a group wield considerable power, but they do take issue with Spender's account of the extent to which men consciously use it in a coercive fashion. They suggest that many of the things that continue to maintain unequal relationships between men and women are not consciously constructed. They believe that patterns of socialization, child rearing and social discourse all replicate these inequalities in more subtle ways. The implication is that, while much of the disadvantage suffered by women derives from the intended and unintended actions of men, it is also maintained by the behaviour of women (Davis, 1991). Cameron (1992) also, takes issue with the passive and overly-determined conception of women implicit within Spender's account. Both point out that, despite the real power that men have over the bastions of education and the media, that women have always used language too. That is, that there are many situations in which women have some capacity to decide how they speak, and what they speak about. Both Cameron and Davis, see the power of language as a dynamic one, that is, while it is to some degree presented ready-made to the speaker, it is also made or unmade each time that it is used.

Nevertheless, Cameron (1992) agrees that language is used as a form of social control of women. In discussing the language of insults, she states that 'the derogation of women reflects a reality in which men regard us as inferior and define us as above all in terms of our sexual attributes'. Like Lees (1986), she notes that women themselves, play a critical role in this process of control, by carefully monitoring their own behaviour to avoid negative labels like 'slag' and 'slut' and also by policing the behaviour of other women.

POWER IN PRACTICE

The interaction between the helper and the helped, the unhealthy and the healthy, and the poor and the not-poor, occurs in circumstances in which the existing bases of power such as knowledge, wealth, expertise, resources and status are mediated through language. It is in the communication between the two parties that each has some opportunity to create or re-create their power and influence, or to challenge it. It is within the immediate relationship that the micro-level features of communication reviewed earlier in this chapter are displayed. Within the social microcosm of their relationship, participants may confirm the existing order and challenge or create, however fleetingly, a new one. While the exercise of physical force, economic power and legal stricture are, *in extremis*, undoubtedly central to the maintenance of social order, it is the everyday mundane creation and re-creation of meaning that does much to preserve it.

Language is at the crux of health and welfare practice, because it constructs the internal subjective world of each participant and acts as a bridge between the individual and the 'external' social world. We should recognize that many of the prevailing discourses within current practice are disadvantageous to our clients. Oliver (1990), in his discussion of the discourse of disability, argues that, despite the rhetoric which has seen a shift from the word 'client' to 'consumer', the relationship between professionals and people with disability is still one that creates and sustains dependency. For example, the professional definition of independence often revolves around the acquisition of daily living skills such as washing, dressing, cooking, and so on, whereas the person with a disability is much more likely to see independence as about being in control of the decisions within one's life (Taylor, 1993).

A recognition of the multiplicity of subjective experience implies that we can rarely assume a congruence of meaning and purpose between the worker and the client. The consequences of this are not limited simply to problems of misunderstanding for, in a situation where one person is more powerful than another, it is probable that that person's views will prevail. As Rodger (1991) has noted, 'Failure to empathize with the client's motivations is more likely to lead a social worker to a correctional approach to practice' – that is, an approach in which the problem is presumed to lie within the client. Thus, subsequent intervention is limited solely to individual treatment or adjustment.

CONCLUSION

Within the human services there is a continuing debate about what term to use to describe the people who use the services – 'clients', 'patients', 'residents', 'service users', 'customers', and so on. Such sensitivity to nomenclature indicates the fundamental nature of the question being posed – what is the proper orientation of nurses, doctors and social workers to the public who require their help? The debate may be seen as an attempt to come to terms with the problems raised by the intrinsic disparity of power between the professional and the client. The criticisms aimed at political correctness tend to characterize it as a trivial and humourless debate about terminology, whereas it is more accurately seen as a fundamental question about power – the power to define not so much which words to use but what the words represent or mean.

This chapter proposes that power derives from the potential of language to influence what other people think or do, from the styles and strategies of personal interaction through to the broader macroscopic shaping of the types of knowledge that it is possible to have. This approach proposes that knowledge and meaning are human constructions arising from social actions and can therefore be shaped by intentional and unintentional efforts.

Furthermore, as Kuhn (1970) recognized, much of what is deemed acceptable knowledge is paradigmatic in nature. It is subject to the power of those who are able to reward or ignore the proponents of particular ideas. Through their actions, those with the power of appointment or of publication, or the capacity to exert personal influence, are able to influence the broad discourse, that is, the ideas and meanings we hold about the world – and thus ultimately to shape the way in which we act in the world. We should remind ourselves that the ideas that we have about the world are not always consciously acquired or replicated. The power of language is not always intentionally manipulated: the replication of discrimination and oppression arises as much from the taken-for-granted nature of language as from the deliberate subjugation of other people. For example, the pervasive power of racism is established and reinforced by the implicit frames of reference embodied within everyday speech and thought. It is the dehumanizing ideas espoused by the perpetrators, which objectify or reify the other person from a human being into 'thing' status, which legitimize within their own minds their sometimes murderous and disfiguring behaviour.

Similarly, the disabling effects of physical impairment arise not simply from the impairments but from the social response to them. For example, the prevailing model for comprehending disability is a medical model, that is, an approach that seeks to explain disability in terms of the aetiology of the impairment and understand it in terms of the resulting deficiency or loss of capacity (Swain et al., 1993). This model tends to ignore the most significant aspect of disability, which is that the handicap that the disabled person experiences derives largely from the social reactions to impairment, which lead to poverty from lack of employment and isolation from lack of transport, and the damaging effects of low self-esteem, which derive from the perception of difference as abnormality and impairment as tragedy. This limited model, which conceptualizes impairment as a form of individual pathology and ignores virtually all the social aspects of disability, is uncritically reproduced and reiterated by health professionals, who continue to describe people in terms of their illness or 'incapacity': 'amputees', 'schizophrenics', 'diabetics', 'CVAs', 'mentally handicapped', and so on.

This chapter set out to raise awareness of how language may represent power and be used to create it. My purpose was to encourage a conscious awareness of the potential of language within our work. As the earlier discussion on the consequences of language definition indicated, there is little doubt that those who plan, organize and deliver health and social services are, for whatever reasons, abusing the power that they wield. It is possible that it is ignorance and unconscious linguistic prejudice, rather than informed deliberation, which results in the disenfranchisement of many minority groups from much needed health and welfare services. However, as we shall see in Chapter 7, permanent ignorance of the needs of relatively powerless and marginalized groups is simply unacceptable within an explicit antidiscriminatory approach to practice.

Language and theory

Philosophers have only interpreted the world, in various ways; the point is to change it.

Marx, cited in McLellan, 1975

INTRODUCTION

This chapter reviews the extent to which some of the popular and well established theories used in nursing and social work provide a satisfactory account of language, culture and power.

The first two sections of this chapter review the current position of nursing and social work theory, and proposes that they are deficient in their consideration of language issues. The third and fourth sections review counselling and communication theory, because these are often used to underpin practice. My conclusion is that, while some progress is being made, most current theory could be described as **alinguistic**, because of the tendency to take language for granted and thus omit its critical role in establishing identity and creating and sustaining power.

Nursing and social work have both been described as semi-professions, that is, occupations whose work, organization and status have some of the features of the established professions like law and medicine. These professions supposedly have a high degree of professional autonomy, especially in controlling entry to the profession, and also claim to have special knowledge and skills. Both nursing and social work have made claim to distinctive formal knowledge and have striven to establish their credibility in this respect, but neither have been able to establish the levels of prestige and remuneration attached to professions such as law and medicine. Within each field there is a variety of theoretical knowledge, much of which is relatively modest in its range, in that it does not attempt to establish grand theories which encompass low and high level phenomena. Most of this formal knowledge does not even claim the status of formal theory, but rather, is aimed at establishing effective models for intervention and is thus less concerned with underpinning theories of human action or explanations of cause and effect.

For a number of reasons, most social work theorists have abandoned the search for unified grand theories of professional practice. This partly derives from the influence of sociology, which has provided a continuously critical academic base. For example, the popularity of systems theory has waned as the limitations of the approach became apparent (Langan, 1993). It was seen to be overly abstract and often uncritical in its problem focus and, while professing to acknowledge wider structural forces, in practice the actual interventions remained largely focused upon the individual person. The diversity of social work has also obstructed the attempts at unification (Clarke, 1993).

Additionally, there has been a growing pessimism about the potential of social work, fuelled in part by the widely publicized inquiries into the mismanagement of child care and protection (Langan, 1993). Within social work, scepticism about the pursuit of professionalism is exemplified in the following quotation: 'The desperate attempt to make social work a repository of detailed scientific knowledge is desensitizing us in the unworthy cause of professional legitimation' (Simpkin, 1979). This disillusionment and retrenchment from the more optimistic visions of what social work might accomplish, was aptly described by Simpkin (1979) as 'the pricking of the social work bubble'. The succession of Government-funded enquiries into the nature and purpose of social work have further reinforced an atmosphere of uncertainty and doubt (Bamford, 1990).

Nursing, meanwhile, has suffered fewer occupational traumas and there is, arguably, a more optimistic professional outlook. The academic base of nursing has been strengthened by the development of the graduate qualification and the accompanying expansion of university and college lecturing staff. The professional literature is extensive and expanding, and the position of nursing is rarely criticized outside the profession. The formal knowledge base remains strongly linked to medicine, and the impact of the social sciences, though growing, has been more limited and is more recent. Consequently, unlike social work, there has not been a professional denouement: professional confidence remains relatively high. The following discussion of language in nursing theory reflects my perception that generally there has been a less critical approach within some areas of nursing knowledge. The fact that the discussion is more critical of nursing than social work is not intended to proclaim the superiority of the latter over the former, but is a reflection of the different circumstances of each occupational group. As Owen and Holmes (1993) suggest, 'nursing has only just begun to explore its conceptual and epistemological possibilities'.

NURSING THEORY

Since the 1960s nursing theorists have considerably developed the scope of nursing theory beyond a simple patient-focused or pathological model. During the last 30 years, many writers and academics have adopted a new approach to training, an approach that has been characterized as a shift from an apprentice-ship model, which emphasized learning on the job and vocational skills, towards a professional model, which emphasizes the creation of a distinctive body of nursing knowledge and practice (Leddy and Pepper, 1993). While it should be acknowledged that not all writers agree with this shift (Melosh, 1982), the nursing literature has enthusiastically adopted professionalism and the accompanying expansion of nursing knowledge. Important elements of this 'new knowledge' can be seen in the distinction between endogenous factors of health, that is, those that arise from the patient, and exogenous factors, that is, those that are external to the patient (Leddy and Pepper, 1993). There has also been a recognition of transcultural factors of health (Leininger, 1967, 1978; Wilkins, 1993), and a more enveloping conceptualization of health in the holistic approaches (Flynn, 1980). This 'new knowledge' encompasses two important perceptions:

- that the patient is not a passive person but an active one;
- that the context in which the patient and nursing are situated is wider than the immediate physical surroundings: that it is a social and cultural environment.

This approach is in distinct contrast to earlier theorists, who tended to assume a passive patient to whom things would be done by medical personnel. The task of training was therefore to develop the expertise of nurses to complement the technical skills of doctors. In so far as the patient had needs, they were assumed to be universal and fairly limited. The environment, that is, the situation and the world external to the immediate medical setting, were considered narrowly, and only to the extent that they contributed to pathology, for example, sanitation, prevention of cross infection, and so on. In the new approaches to understanding health, especially those described as holistic, the person is not simply regarded as a technical/medical problem passively awaiting treatment and care, but someone who has a social, intellectual and psychological life too. Thus the mind/body separation characteristic of the earlier pathological model has been rejected as being simplistic and ineffective. Holistic approaches to nursing typically conceptualize **wellness** as being more than the avoidance of illness or pain: health is seen as a more embracing notion. Thus holistic theorists are critical of current medical practice, which they perceive as being, ultimately, reductionist in its narrow focus upon symptoms and diagnosis. Similarly, the idea that nursing care takes place in a social and cultural vacuum has been modified or explicitly rejected, since both the patient and the carer are, to some extent, viewed as being both unique individuals and to some degree, the products or carriers of specific social and cultural environments.

While there is theoretical debate about whether holism represents simply the recognition of these wider factors or is a more thoroughgoing attempt to avoid the perils of reductionism, especially in an acknowledgement of spiritual and psychological dimensions (Flynn, 1980; Owen and Holmes, 1993), the overall shift towards a professional stance has been quite remarkable in opening up the range of theoretical debate within nursing. Increasingly, nursing textbooks include discussion of the philosophical bases of theory and research, as well as the usual descriptions of nursing theories. The need to socialize the novice professional is widely acknowledged and great stress is laid upon the importance of developing reflective practitioners who, it is intended, will become sophisticated, critical users and creators of knowledge. This is a far cry from the narrowly focused days of routine work on the ward, of beds and baths, 'doctor knows best' and autocratic ward sisters (Porter, 1994). Within this broader conception of nursing knowledge, there is frequent reference to communication skills and the use of language. There is also a widespread acceptance of the possibility of cultural misunderstanding between patient and nurse. The increasing theoretical sophistication of nursing has been broadly welcomed by nursing trainers and academics, though latterly there is some scepticism about the motivation for this, which, Porter (1994) states, 'seems to have as much to do with the prospect of an improved occupational status for nursing as it has to do with nurses' altruistic desires to improve the lot of their patients'.

A CRITIQUE OF NURSING THEORY

This section provides a critique of this new knowledge and suggests that most theorists are only making notional reference to language; that for the most part their work contains little discussion of the central issue of power, and very little consideration of the role of language in creating and sustaining power within health care services. Of course, as noted earlier, it would be facile to aim these criticisms at the majority of low-level theories, which do not attempt to provide encompassing explanations of nursing. Instead, they are aimed at those approaches that seek to establish 'grand' theories.

Unfortunately, the holistic approaches to nursing theory that appear to hold the greatest prospect of a sustained consideration of power and language, upon closer examination reveal themselves to be seriously flawed. There is confusion about what holism actually means (Owen and Holmes, 1993). Most accounts, rather than being inclusive and encompassing, are characterized by serious omissions in their models and explanations of nursing (Bruni, 1989; Williams, 1989). The term **system** is often used without clear definition (Phillips, 1977), and theorists often use description as if it constituted explanation (Deising, 1971). Few holists tackle the important questions about epistemology and ontology raised by their approach to knowledge. That is, they fail to answer the questions about what it is possible to know and what the status is of what we think we know. For example, holistic writers argue that reductionism fails to capture the totality of experience and phenomena but, as we saw in the earlier discussion in Chapters 1 and 4, it is arguable that some degree of reductionism is inevitable in human thought. Language and the mental categories which it constructs will always be typifications that are, to some extent, simplifications of the world. Words are always symbolic representations and not the things that they signify. How can it be otherwise?

While holism, in its unifying conception of 'wholeness', has been strongly influenced by Eastern traditions of thought, in its humanistic assumptions it is guilty of uncritically representing personal growth as a universal goal. It seems unable to understand how this idea is, in essence, an ethnocentric Western conception of the self. While it recognizes the potential conflict between cultures, it does not recognize that the idea of an impulse to seek growth may be inherently culturally bound (Saleh, 1989). Thus, holistic approaches can be criticized for the tendency to embrace the broader aspects of the social world only in so far as they are directly represented in the constitution of the individual. While they may acknowledge the political and social aspects of a situation, they tend to ignore the ways in which these things affect the individual's present state. Writers like Orem (1985) and Blattner (1981) discuss health as if it were contingent solely upon the choices made by free individuals. They almost completely ignore the extent to which broader structural factors such as class, gender, age and ethnicity impinge upon people, let alone consider how personal choice may be structured by these factors. Thus in regard to the issue of power, holistic approaches seem unaware of how their own discourse shapes thinking about health in a way that frequently assigns total responsibility, if not causality, to the individual.

The end result is a form of understanding that offers only a limited and depoliticized view of health problems and health. It is as if they have failed to follow through the implications of the more embracing holistic conceptions and have stayed on safe ground, avoiding the dangerous territory of medical power and political analysis. Much of the supposed inclusiveness and wholeness of holistic theory is empty rhetoric, which leads Owen and Holmes (1993) to conclude that it 'should be regarded as an essentially conservative philosophy which works within the status quo rather than challenging it'. Holism, in most of its writings, ultimately represents a romanticization of individualism, divorced from the political and social factors which affect the quality of people's lives.

Within much of the 'new nursing' (Porter, 1994), there has been a recognition of the intersubjectivity of meaning, that is, an acknowledgement that different people have different meanings; that what is meant by words and phrases is often variable, shifting and sometimes elusive. Consequently, in some of the popular nursing texts such as Chinn and Kramer (1991), there has been great stress placed upon the importance of defining concepts and clarifying meaning. Clearly, this is vital if misunderstandings are to be avoided. A nursing colleague recently recounted an incident in which a doctor, upon completing his examination of a patient who was dying of cancer, prescribed 'TLC' (tender loving care). She, to the embarrassment of her colleagues, asked him what he meant by this. Did it mean, for example that a Ryles tube should be used to avoid dehydration? The doctor's response in an exasperated tone of voice, was predictable: 'You know what it means!' As she persevered in her attempt to seek clarification of what **he** meant, the doctor became angry and frustrated with her and eventually stormed off, only to return later and, to his credit, concede that he did not know exactly what he meant by the term. They then agreed upon what should be done and both acknowledged that this term, which seemed to be a matter of 'common sense', had considerable potential for misunderstanding.

Chinn and Kramer (1991), in the preface of their popular textbook, have explicitly attempted to simply and clarify their own language and they note that, as:

> we became aware of more 'flaws' in the underlying structure of the language and tried to address them as consistently as possible. We became conscious of value assumptions and connotations that were inherent in the language. Many of the terms that are commonly associated with the practice of scientific methods carry antagonistic, adversarial, objectifying and militaristic connotations that are contrary to the ethic of caring... we sought to shift the language to words that carry a similar literal meaning but a more human and caring value connotation. For example, instead of the phrase 'argue your position,' we use instead 'share your ideas'.
>
> *Chinn and Kramer, 1991*

However, 'to argue your position' implies an awareness of potential difference or conflict of views, and perhaps more accurately represents the structuring of knowledge, whereby some people's views, by dint of their formal position or conversational competence, carry more weight than others. Of course, the phrase 'share your ideas' reflects an admirable intention – to recognize the validity of the other person's perspective – but it also obscures the fact of existing inequalities in power and position. Apart from the issue of intention, it is doubtful whether the two phrases do actually convey the same meaning to most people. Nevertheless, Chinn and Kramer believe that 'the shifts in the language are profound', because they usher in a new era in nursing, where the nursing student is empowered and engaged directly by the active style of language and the avoidance of a prescriptive approach.

There are serious omissions in their book. There is no substantive discussion of how language carries or constructs meaning, nor of related concepts such as power and culture. This is surprising, given the earlier awareness in the preface. Like many popular texts, their work contains no reference to language, culture or power in the glossary and has little or no reference to these factors in the index. It is arguable that even the conscious shift in their own use of language, exemplified in the above quotation, depoliticizes knowledge. Further evidence of muddled thinking about language is shown in the brief discussion on words, ideas and their meanings. Chinn and Kramer state that the meaning of any idea is derived from the interaction of three forms of experience, '1) the word or other symbolic label, 2) the thing itself (object, property or event), and 3) feelings, values and attitudes associated with the word and with the perception of the material thing'. Thus, people's ideas of a word like 'mother' are shaped in part by their contact 'with an actual person', but 'at the same time, the human meaning of the concept "mother" is formed from cultural and societal heritages that all people of a culture share, regardless of individual experiences in early childhood'.

At first glance, this seems both probable and logical, but there are some problems here. First, what is culture? At the social level, they do not define what a culture is. Is it something shared by all people in a given nation, or is there a plurality of cultures within most societies? From reading the rest of the text, it is unlikely that they presume a single homogeneous culture shared by all people in a given society, since this is manifestly mistaken. Most probably, they presume cultural diversity within a given society, but the difficulty here is that neither similarities nor differences of meaning are restricted to differences between cultural groups. For example, as many feminist writers have noted, the patriarchal ideas held about women span different cultural groups; thus the social meaning of the word 'mother' may be structured more by gender than culture. It is ironic that the proponents of conceptual clarity should ignore their own prescriptions and assume that we share a common understanding of the meaning of culture. As Garfinkel (1967) has demonstrated, closer examination of such 'common sense' often reveals considerable ambiguity.

Similar difficulties with the concept of culture appear in the work of Leddy and Pepper (1993). They cite Leininger (1967) in support of their view that 'Each cultural group has a special pattern of living and interacting together', which is maintained by the norms that regulate behaviour. These are 'the stable rules of behaviour that prescribe the behaviour to be followed, and they tend to consciously and unconsciously regulate our lives and help us solve many life problems'. This approach is problematic in two ways. First, it presents norms as if they were stable entities that exist outside of our behaviour, whereas a more accurate conceptualization might be that it is our language and behaviour that represent and reiterate these social rules. Social norms may well be the product of other people's behaviour, and thus we may be recipients of these received rules, but we are not passive recipients: we have the potential to accept, reject or alter these impositions. As we saw in Chapter 5, we are neither wholly determined nor wholly free; our interaction with our social world is far more complex and ambiguous. Second, Leddy and Pepper uncritically represent these social norms as positive features of social life. They may well be necessary elements, but to assume that their effects are invariably positive, especially with regard to norms about health, is clearly mistaken. For example, the stoicism with which many working-class men endure life-threatening ailments without seeking treatment can be seen as a highly risky social norm.

Some nursing theorists seem unable to see that their theories and the language with which they describe them are likely to be alienating to both student practitioners and patients. For example, Barrett (1989), in a discussion of power in which she uses Martha Rogers's theory, blithely uses sentences such as: 'Consistent with the Rogerian building blocks of energy fields, openness, pattern, and four-dimensionality, power was defined as the capacity to participate knowingly in the nature of change characterizing the continuous, innovative patterning of the human and environmental fields', and, later on the same page, 'Human field motion is an experience of process, change, and wave frequency that is postulated to transcend time and space as well as movement and stillness'! The notion that nurses should engage their clients in a mutually educative process using such quasi-mystical conceptualizations seems quite bizarre. Far from enhancing communication and understanding, they are more likely to obstruct it. These attempts to marry analytical models derived from physics with the self-actualizing tenets of person-centred approaches to care do little to promote effective practice. Fortunately, there is a wide gulf between theory and practice in this respect. Such theories probably do more to promote the power of the exponents of the new paradigm rather than enhance that of the patients. Despite their disclaimers to the contrary, these theorists may unwittingly become 'experts' who explain to the uninitiated how to act and understand the world, which is the very role they ostensibly have sought to avoid.

What is apparent in their work is an insufficiently developed model of the person in the social world. This approach therefore, tends not to explore the links between micro and macro levels of culture and the role of language. With the exception of the occasional reference to gender and feminism, or 'race' and ethnicity, it largely ignores other significant dimensions of difference, such as age, class and sexuality. The cultural meanings attached to these different dimensions may be structured across a whole society and not simply be held by particular groups within it. Thus, there is a need for a broader structural analysis of meaning, because, for example, patriarchal ideas are rarely espoused by one group alone. Furthermore, with a few exceptions (Hewison, 1994), the concept of power is often unexplored, or is treated superficially without reference to more recent theoretical developments. The uncritical representation of power can be seen in the manner in which they implicitly accept certain political ideas. For example, Leddy and Pepper (1993), in a discussion of health care changes, suggest that the funding problem facing US health care arises from 'high physician fees... encouraged by lack of competitive pressures'. They simply ignore alternative explanations, such as the idea that it might arise from a lack of government control or from exploitation of competitive advantage. Thus, the context of health care is depoliticized by a limited consideration of the causes and responses to problems.

The implicit functionalism which pervades much nursing theory is virtually identical to the representations of power utilized in many sociological theories in the 1960s. Society is presented as a pluralistic structure in which ordered discussion and reason generally prevail. Conflict is minimized and perceived as dysfunctional because it distracts from the orderly working of society. This is a Utopian portrayal of society – a *Candide*-like view of it, as the best of all possible worlds – whereby some people have more money and power and better jobs for the simple reason that they are the best at those things, and thus are deserving of them. The uncritical acceptance of 'things as they are' leads to a circular form of reasoning which can also be found within many linguistic theories. The limitations of such assumptions have been trenchantly criticized by Williams (1992). To avoid offering an analysis of power is not to remain neutral but to sustain the status quo through an unquestioning acceptance of things as they are. Thus, some of the significant developments in theories of power, such as the idea that words and meanings are representations of social structure and that it is their creation and reiteration which constructs that structure, are absent.

The consequence of this omission of power is a rather ambiguous type of theory, in which the issue of how individuals use language to think and construct meanings is a curiously disengaged and depoliticized process. They have opened up their theories to an appreciation of the patient's subjective appreciation of her/his experience, and though some writers clearly see power as an issue, they have not opened them up sufficiently. Acceptance of the relevance of power typically remains at a superficial level. For example, Raatikainen (1994) suggests that powerful people not only have good self-image and motivation, but almost invariably have a deep moral awareness and are empathetic and respectful of others. These qualities are linked without any convincing explanation. Consequently, power is presented positively, as if it cannot be abused or misused. Many writers, like Leddy and Pepper (1993), identify different forms or sources of power, but then fail to use or develop these within their subsequent analysis. However, what is most surprising is the relative paucity of substantive discussion of how meaning is constructed and the role of common sense in everyday professional life. Almost no reference is made to the work of the conversation analysts, let alone the research into power and influence. One might suspect that the adoption of the hermeneutic/phenomenological perspective as a form of research (Benner, 1985; Omery, 1983), which recognizes the importance of the person's subjective experience, is legitimated by the fact that, used narrowly, it is unlikely to threaten the implicitly assumed consensus on power.

Other theorists who explicitly tackle power also do it in ways that are problematic. The theories of Rogers, mentioned earlier, have spawned a literature rich in obfuscation. For example, 'Power is a noncausal phenomenon. It is helpful for clients to recognize that neither they nor the environment control anything' (Barrett, 1989). Who and what is this environment? Here it appears to be presented as some mysterious dimension, but surely the consequences of power are available for examination. When nurses deliberately do harm to their patients, when doctors are overworked, when resource constraints result in diminished services to patients, all of these things have identifiable consequences. In a philosophical sense this statement about power may be arguable, but it ignores the subjective reality, which is that most people attach a degree of causality to their actions and those of other people too. Furthermore, this statement, far from enabling the nurse and patient, is more likely to be disempowering in its consequences.

There are four main areas of criticism of nursing theory.

- Theorists fail to follow their own prescriptions on language – for example, the uncritical use of generic male pronouns for clients and the female equivalents for nurses. They also fail to adequately define key concepts, such as culture.
- There is an uncritical representation of theories and concepts, such as power and 'race' (Chinn and Kramer, 1991). For example, accounts of Rogers's work (1970, 1988) fail to comment upon its abstract reifications or its propensity to mystification.
- There is an inadequate model of the person in society.
- Most texts offer little sustained consideration of the role of language and power.

The result is a curiously free-floating body of writing which, especially in the textbooks, creates the impression that one can simply choose and use any theory one likes. In many instances, there is little discussion of the practical implications which follow from the use of a particular theory. Problems of validity and eclecticism are skimmed over in many of the 'grand texts'. Nursing theory often presents a disembodied, depoliticized world, which is all the more surprising since so many of their writers seem to be aware of the potential pitfalls. Surely acceptance of the subjectivity of phenomena should necessitate a more detailed discussion of meaning and how it is constructed and represented?

Fortunately, the 'grand textbooks' do not represent the totality of nursing theory and within the journals at least there is a burgeoning interest in linguistic issues. There have been some interesting developments in exploring the ways in which language creates and sustains particular ideas about nursing. Discourse analysis is becoming more popular, and Owen and Holmes (1993) have provided an interesting account of how 'holism' has become a rather quixotic term within nursing theory. Phillips (1993) has deconstructed the term 'caring', and shown how fallacious distinctions between physical and emotional care have hindered the development of 'a truly psychotherapeutic role for psychiatric nurses'. Czechmeister (1994), following on from the work of Sontag (1978), has explored the implications of the use of metaphor in nursing and nurse education and concludes that 'in the light of the shift towards an interpretive paradigm in ... nursing, metaphor has been shown to be a valuable gateway into the perceptual world of others, particularly those facing the crisis of illness'.

Nevertheless, apart from discussion about the identity of nursing itself, there is still relatively little general exploration of the role of language in constructing identity. One interesting exception, by Baker, Arseneault and Gallant (1994), examines the resettlement experience of culturally isolated migrants. The study confirmed the sense of discontinuity that was experienced by the migrants and noted a common phenomenon of marginalization – a sense of heightened awareness and sensitivity towards other people.

SOCIAL WORK THEORY

Earlier, I noted that social work theory appeared to be less ambitious than nursing theory and this doubtless created the impression that there were fewer problems with it. Certainly, social work theory appears to avoid most of the more obvious criticisms made of nursing theory, simply because most social work academics have abandoned ambitious attempts to create 'grand theory' for their profession. Their work is not only less ambitious in scope but also, arguably, more grounded in the traditions of psychology and sociology. Thus theorists are generally ready to accept the epistemological uncertainty arising from the acknowledgement of multiple paradigms and discourses of knowledge. In contrast, some contributors to nursing knowledge resist this: for example, Sharp (1994) argues that it is inappropriate for such an action-oriented practice as nursing. While Sharp's views may not be representative, this stance probably echoes the views of many nurse practitioners, who believe that training is becoming overly theoretical. However, despite avoiding some of the bigger pitfalls, social work theory contains many similar problems with regard to issues of language.

The dominant trend in the formal knowledge of contemporary social work is a recognition of the problems of marginalization and disadvantage. This, of course, is no surprise, since social workers have always been involved with the administration of welfare to the poorest groups within society, and problems of poverty and lack of resources still remain significant dimensions in their work. In this respect, social work practitioners have long accepted a form of social holism. Even the founders of the Charity Organization Society (1869) acknowledged the limits of social casework. Richmond (1917, 1922), the first formal theorist of casework, recognized its limits and accepted that other methods of intervention, such as groupwork, social action and reform, might be required. In the immediate post-Second-World-War period, Pray (1949) wrote that social work was involved with: 'helping individuals meet the problems of their constantly shifting relations with one another and with the whole society, and to helping the whole society, at the same time, adjust its demands upon its members and its services to them in accordance with the real needs of the individuals that compose and determine its life'.

However, acceptance of the possibility that people's problems were not always pathological, in the sense that the root causes lay beyond the immediate situation, was tempered by an awareness of the limits of social work. Smalley (1967) was typical in her view that 'social work is in danger of taking unto itself a too total responsibility for the cause and cure of social problems in a way that ignores their complexity, the many factors that enter into their genesis, and the many professional disciplines as well as the will of the body politic which must enter into their resolution or alleviation'.

The formal knowledge of social work has from its earliest days encompassed a debate about what the proper focus of social work should be, together with an accompanying concern about the politicization of workers (Simpkin, 1979; Davies, 1985). Perhaps what is most distinctive about the contemporary focus is:

- a recognition of socially structured forms of disadvantage based upon such factors as age, disability, ethnicity, gender and sexuality;
- a developing professional awareness by social workers that their work is not automatically beneficial in its consequences: that they might be part of the problem, not the solution;
- the emphasis, at least formally, on a needs-led approach to the provision of service, that is, one in which the service providers attempt to be responsive to the particular problems of the client rather than one in which the client simply has to accept what is available.

The first point does not mean that social workers do not recognize the possibility that some people create their own problems. It has, for example, become axiomatic in assessing the practical competence of trainees to consider their knowledge of such structural factors. The second point refers to the increased awareness that social work itself may have deleterious consequences for the most vulnerable people in society, that the actions of social workers may unwittingly reinforce and contribute to social disadvantage. These three points are currently embodied within the **antidiscriminatory perspective**, which has become one of the touchstones of modern social work practice, along with 'community care' and 'needs-led service'. It is all the more surprising, therefore, to find that consideration of the role of language in the construction of attitude, identity and power within contemporary social work theory and practice, is with few exceptions, largely superficial.

The legitimacy of antidiscriminatory practice is not yet fully established within social work practice. But it is firmly ensconced within the formal knowledge base (Davis and Proctor, 1989; Dominelli, 1988; Thompson, 1993) and, despite efforts to diminish its significance, it continues to be promoted by the Central Council for Education and Training in Social Work in the UK and, in a less paradigmatic fashion, by the National Association of Social Workers in the USA. Antidiscriminatory theory begins with the recognition that 'certain actions, attitudes and structures have the effect of oppressing particular individuals and groups' (Thompson, 1993), and that this oppression is maintained by the intended and unintended consequences of the actions of those with power, and also by the incorporation of oppressive ideologies into the thinking of both oppressors and oppressed.

This approach acknowledges many dimensions of discrimination within society, which are typically located around demographic differences such as age, class, ethnicity and gender, but also include disability and sexual orientation. The extent to which these factors are experienced positively or negatively by individuals largely depends upon how those who have power think and act towards those whom they perceive to be different from them. The chances of discrimination and the consequent disadvantage which arises from it are socially structured, in the sense that the point of location on these multiple dimensions is predictive of the experience of a group, if not of any particular person within that group. For example, while class background may be highly predictive of health and wealth chances for a group, it is not necessarily so for any given individual member, who by dint of good fortune, or their own actions, may avoid or escape the possible consequences of membership.

The interaction of these demographic factors is highly complex and, while the fact of, say, black skin in a predominantly white society is probably a good indicator of potential life experience, other factors such as class and gender will also play their part in determining actual experience. As Dominelli (1988) states, 'the intertwining [sic] of class and race differentiates black people's experience of class oppression from white people's'. The antidiscriminatory perspective recognizes the possibility of multiple oppression and, though it accepts a high degree of determinism in terms of group chances, it crucially avoids an overly determined view of the individual. Thus individuals do have some freedom to think and act. The implication for professionals who possess power is that they can make a difference, they may choose to ignore discrimination or attempt to reduce it. Service users, too, have some capacity for willed action and planned change and, consequently, they do not have to submit totally to the actions of the workers who serve them, nor to a fatalistic acceptance of the limitations of their immediate circumstances.

A CRITIQUE OF SOCIAL WORK THEORY

The antidiscriminatory paradigm, as noted earlier, is not yet fully accepted or fully developed, despite the abandonment of earlier attempts to develop antioppressive practice, which adopted the counterproductive forms of 'race awareness training'. There are still some people who refuse to accept a dynamic approach to this knowledge and consequently misuse the antidiscriminatory perspective as a means of furthering their own power. Rather than accept that this is an area in which practice and theory are developing rapidly, they dogmatically use the new knowledge to establish their own superiority. This is apparent in the way in which the language of antidiscriminatory practice is often misunderstood, trivialized or made problematic in irrelevant ways. A student recently recounted an incident which occurred on her practice placement. She had offered to make coffee at a meeting and upon asking whether people wanted it 'black or white' (i.e. with or without milk) was sternly reprimanded for using 'racist' language. From the point of view of antidiscriminatory practice, as we shall see in the concluding chapter, the main test of an action lies in its consequences – will it empower or disempower the recipient? In this instance, the words 'black' and 'white' are not being used with any intention of reinforcing negative or positive connotations, nor do they do so in practice. Their descriptive significance is clear and unambiguous. Of course, the consequences of using 'black' as a negative descriptor are widely recognized; thus it would be deemed discriminatory to use terms like 'blackmail', 'blackguard' and 'blackball', because these specifically carry a negative connotation which derogates the word 'black' and by reference anything else to which it is applied, such as black people. Whether the negative connotation arises from discriminatory notions about black people or from other ideas, such as day and night, has become irrelevant, for their significance is now widely understood as a racist slur.

Within the literature upon antidiscriminatory practice there is, not surprisingly, reference to language and its representations. However, this rarely ventures beyond the level of prescriptions for practice – for example, exhortations to avoid using words that represent negative stereotypes of people. While this is clearly relevant, it nevertheless is an insufficient analysis, because typically it fails to spell out how and why changing language might make a difference. Obviously, in the context of any helping relationship, the use of words and phrases that the service user regards as insulting or offensive is likely to hinder communication and impede effective practice. The service user might well conclude that the worker was either insensitive or ignorant of the implications of the ill-chosen language they had used. In either case it is unlikely to inspire confidence. It would be hypocritical if the purpose of avoiding such language were solely to avoid giving offence; there must be some underpinning assumption about how words construct meaning and social reality, since it is obvious that merely mouthing the 'politically correct' language does not ensure understanding and acceptance of the precepts of enlightened practice. It is in this respect that much of social work theory is deficient, because its reference to language is primarily concerned with attitudes and communication, it tends to ignore other aspects such as meaning and how language interacts with identity and power. Language is often a taken-for-granted element in social work theory, which tends to assume a rather static quality to it. Therefore, while there may be a struggle to avoid labelling and negative stereotyping, little consideration is given to the issue of whether the language constructs the social reality, reflects it, or does both.

At the heart of most writing on antidiscriminatory practice is the proposal that social workers should become **conscientized** (Chapter 2). This task as envisaged by Dominelli, begins with the familiar Socratic injunction to 'know thyself', not simply in terms of one's emotions, attitudes and values but in the sociological and political sense too – that is, within the context of the workplace, the organization and the wider society. In the case of racism, Dominelli usefully identifies a variety of strategies that white people use to avoid confronting the difficult issues it raises. Among these strategies is **decontextualization**, which is defined as an acceptance that racism 'exists in general terms', but an unawareness of how it 'permeates everyday activities'. This decontextualization is explored primarily in terms of the implicit assumptions used by workers, which disadvantage black service users. For example, the assumption that black people's problems are the same as white people's except that they have more of them. This assumption ignores the fact that not only is it white workers, in the main, who are administering casework to black people, but that the experience of black people which precedes contact with social workers is different. This experience typically includes overt racism and hostility and may also encompass feelings of low self-esteem and worthlessness.

Unfortunately, while Dominelli states that 'although only one part of it, language is an important aspect of the oppression process', and accurately identifies many examples of implicitly racist assumptions, she does not substantively analyse the role that language plays in both constructing and carrying racism. Central concepts such as culture, ethnicity and ideology are not explicitly defined. Apart from the briefest of references to the work of Spender (1980), no theoretical account of language is offered, nor are the limitations of Spender's determinism acknowledged (see the critique in Chapter 5). Like many writers, Dominelli recognizes some of the pitfalls of communication between people whose languages differ, particularly in the use of unskilled, insensitive and inappropriate translators (Ahmed, 1978; Ely and Denney, 1987), but she does not sufficiently explore the role of language in constructing attitudes, identity and meaning. Though Dominelli refers to the reclamation of language, that is, the recovery and redefinition of words with negative connotations, so that they have new, positive meanings, for example the word 'black', she does not develop this analysis. How is it possible to do this? In what circumstances can reclamation succeed? How is power revealed, created and sustained by language?

In contrast, Thompson's (1993) account of discrimination explicitly links language to the creation of stereotypes and explains how the derogation of other people is accomplished by reducing them to the non-human status of things or objects. Thus language may depersonalize others who are different in some way, for example 'spastic', 'geriatric', and so on. Thompson explores the issue of meaning and representation further by reference to the work of Foucault (1977, 1979) and the concept of discourse. He states that 'discriminatory language therefore both reflects the discriminatory culture and social structure in which we live, and also contributes to the continuance of such discrimination.... The language we use either reinforces discrimination through constructing it as 'normal' or contributes, in some small way at least, to undermining the continuance of a discriminatory discourse.'

The discriminatory discourse of disability, for example by its focus upon physical or mental deficit, contributes to dehumanization, not only through reference to pathology – as in 'amputees', 'brain-damaged', 'wheelchair-bound' – but through the limited perception of the person which it encourages. The continued focus upon the pathology obscures not only the person, but presents this as if it were the only significant or relevant fact about the person. Difference is represented as abnormality and thus, by implication, inferiority (Oliver, 1984, 1990). Furthermore, the typification of those disabled people who manage to get on with their lives as 'heroes/heroines' sustains the notion that self-help and personal motivation are the main features that distinguish them from those disabled people who are not so successful. As Morris states, 'society can abdicate responsibility for collective provision as there is a mostly, but not entirely, unspoken belief that some people just cannot be helped because they are not "survivors" ' (cited in Taylor, 1993).

The other main reason why language is ignored, even within an antidiscriminatory framework is because language nearly always gets subsumed to racial issues. For example, when linguistic difference is noted it is nearly always assumed that there is also racial difference. The assumption is usually that colour is an issue too. This error occurs because of the inadequate conceptualizations employed within much of the writing; many writers continue to use the term 'race' as a synonym for 'colour'. Apart from the fact that race is discredited as a biological category, this leads to two sorts of problem.

- First, it tends to lump all black people together and thus obscures very real differences between ethnic groups.
- Second, it obscures the fact that linguistic variation is not confined to differences between white speakers of English and black speakers of another language.

The first problem arises from a failure to define the terms. Usually there is no attempt to distinguish the term 'black' as a political label from the cultural differences signified by the term 'ethnicity'. The second problem is more common in the British literature, whereas the large number of white and black Spanish speakers in the USA immediately contradicts this mistaken assumption. As Chapters 1 and 2 established, there are many dimensions of linguistic difference as well as many different languages spoken within the UK. Thompson (1993) does not assume that language difference is an issue solely for black people. He recognizes that the imposition of monolingualism is a form of cultural hegemony by which the most powerful groups in society exert their control. This hegemony assumes and promotes the dominance of one language at the expense of others, and thus not only derogates the relatively powerless minority language groups but also operates at the personal level too, so that the personal identity of individuals who are members of the linguistic minorities may also be compromised.

A CRITIQUE OF COUNSELLING THEORY

Counselling theories differ as to the extent to which they are explicitly based upon different theories of communication but, while they embody different styles of communication, all presume some sort of language. Underpinning them is the fundamental premise of symbolic interpersonal communication, that is, communication carried through the words and sounds that symbolize meaning. Most proponents of counselling have sought to increase the linguistic sensitivity of the counsellor, especially in the development of listening skills and also in avoiding the imposition of the counsellor's meaning upon the counsellee's discourse. To different degrees, most approaches to counselling emphasize the skills of sensitive questioning and reflective feedback and seek to establish a climate of acceptance and trust. Within such relationships counsellors are enjoined not to abuse the confidence of the counsellee, nor the power inherent in the relationship. While there has been considerable acknowledgement of the potential problems of interclass and transcultural counselling, relatively few theorists provide any sustained exploration of these issues, two notable exceptions being Sue and Sue (1990) and Davis and Proctor (1989). The major weakness within most counselling theories is that, while they encourage sensitivity to the language and meanings used within the interaction and also recognize the potential for the abuse of power, their analysis of how power is manifested through language is often limited in scope, or in some instances absent.

The major omission arises from the relatively limited focus upon the dyadic (two-person) relationship between the counsellor and counsellee, which tends to exclude or underplay the extent or influence of wider features of language within this relationship. Aspects of language which predate the counselling relationship are played down and it is assumed that these will usually be overcome as the relationship progresses. While this might be possible with variations of accent and dialect, it is manifestly not so for the types of communication style, nor for the form of the discourse itself. Ivey (1981, 1986) has proposed that different types of sentence and meaning are generated not only by different cultures, but by different communication styles too. He suggests that in order to be effective, counsellors should become sensitive to these and develop the ability to shift styles according to the background of the client. However, the prevailing emphasis upon individualism and personal autonomy within counselling theory leads to a 'hands off' approach to the client's problems, problems that may not always arise from their own actions or thoughts (Sue and Sue, 1990) . In the case of ethnic minority counsellees, a more active and influencing style of communication may be a more appropriate approach when the causes lie beyond the individual. Furthermore, the obvious problem with this approach, as Sue and Sue have noted, is that 'style-shift counselling may have personal limitations. We cannot be all things to everyone' (Sue and Sue, 1990). Not only may we have personal limitations upon our capacity to effectively shift styles, we may have difficulty in understanding the counsellee's world view and we may have 'personal biases or racist attitudes that have not been adequately resolved'. The ethnocentricity of most Western counselling theory is also apparent in the humanist presumption of common human needs (Rojek, Peacock and Collins, 1988; Saleh, 1989). As noted earlier in the critiques of nursing theory, the presumption of an impetus to personal growth or optimization contained within most person-centred approaches is by no means universally shared.

A CRITIQUE OF COMMUNICATION THEORY

Some theorists, such as Nelson (1980) and Marcus (1986), have applied communication theory to social work; within this approach human communication is conceptualized as a process of information reception and exchange. 'We perceive the information, and then we evaluate it: this is information processing. As we evaluate communications, we give feedback to the communicator who thus gains some idea of how we have perceived and evaluated the communication' (Payne, 1991). This information is not solely verbal but is composed of many other elements such as kinesis (position and movement), **proxemics** (distance) and **context**. The salient feature of this approach lies in the elucidation of the different patterns or internal 'rules' we develop for processing information, that is, for deciding what to notice and attend to and what to ignore. It is argued that because these internal rules for perception are different, some people are less adept both at deciphering communication from others and in sending out information which other people can understand. This type of problem is often attributed to poor learning. However, information blocks can arise from other internal factors such as intense emotion or direct physical desire for food or sex; they may also arise from external factors such as the patterns of communication established within the communicator's family or wider social group. Communication theory adopts several features of more general systems theory, especially the notion of the inter-relationships of action and effect – the idea that change in one part of a communication system or exchange results in changes elsewhere in the system or exchange.

Communication theory perceptively highlights the importance of feedback in communication and the necessity of consciously evaluating the effectiveness of communication. It has also emphasized the importance of identifying and describing the micro-skills necessary for effective communication. It also purports to locate how and where power is established and maintained within communications. To this end, it offers a conceptual typology that can be used to identify whether relationships are equally balanced or are one-sided and thus, potentially, offers a means of identifying 'gender, ethnic, and other power inequalities' (Payne, 1991). Communications theory, however, suffers from the same sorts of problem as most counselling approaches, in that it tends to focus upon the minutiae of person-to-person communication and fails adequately to explore the external factors sufficiently, or accepts them in an uncritical way. Thus, typically, the focus of intervention remains at the personal level and wider social inequalities are superficially acknowledged in the assessment stage and then largely ignored when it comes to action. In this respect, it repeats the error of the systems and unitary theorists, such as Pincus and Minahan (1973), Goldstein (1973) and Specht and Vickery (1978), whose conceptual framework offered the prospect of a systematic analysis which included the social as well as the personal and thus potentially allowed recognition of structural factors in problem analysis, but then failed in the intervention stage to adopt or deliver the practical implications of the broadened analysis. Typically, such approaches recognize existing inequalities but offer no analysis of how they originate or are sustained (Forder, 1976). This omission effectively depoliticizes people's problems (Webb, 1981; Payne, 1991).

Communications theory, because it is based upon empirical studies of actual conversation, in which how something is communicated is usually more significant than what is communicated, tends to underplay the importance of the actual content of conversation. This is problematic for two reasons. First, it could be argued that, in conversations between service workers and service users, both parties may be more careful about what they say than in more 'normal' conversations. Thus, the content may actually be more significant because they are less likely to rely upon the metalinguistic elements of communication, especially those arising from context. Second, communication analysts, by choosing to focus so extensively upon communication style, are in danger of attributing their own meaning to the other party's dialogue. The parallel with the problem of psychoanalysis is obvious here, because, as Payne (1991) concludes, 'it encourages workers to look for inferred thoughts and problems behind the difficulties expressly presented by clients', while the open nature of the communication, in which the worker is expected to be explicit in feedback about her/his evaluation of the communication as well as her/his understanding of the content, is intended to avoid a double agenda. This remains a real possibility, especially when the user's perspective is misunderstood by the worker or directly challenges the worker's perception of how things are. It is in this respect that the lack of any thoroughgoing analysis of the links between language and culture reveals the approach to be deficient.

CONCLUSION

While the criticisms of holism reveal many problems, it is important to recognize the contribution it has made to nursing theory and not to 'run the risk of throwing the baby out with the bathwater' (Porter, 1994). This contribution is neatly summarized by Owen and Holmes (1993): 'writers in the holist tradition have effectively challenged the positivist tendency to shrink social experiences, such as nursing, until they fit *a priori* categories'. Similarly, while there are clear difficulties with some counselling and communication theories, it is worth noting that it is possible to embrace the skills and some of the constructs of counselling and communication without necessarily promoting these approaches as monolithic explanations of professional interaction and intervention (Burnard, 1989; Lishman, 1994). Some writers adopt some of the models for intervention without necessarily embracing all the accompanying theoretical baggage. While their work is correspondingly more modest in its aims and thus is not as vulnerable to the criticisms made of more formal theory, there are still some problems of omission. Lishman (1994), for example, recognizes that 'the major problems facing social work are those of poverty and discrimination or oppression on the basis of race, class, gender, age and disability', but appears to believe that, while focusing upon communication, these factors can largely be put aside. She acknowledges some limits to her work: 'it is difficult to do justice... to their class, gender, ethnicity, age and personality. In particular, the analysis of communication and culture is limited', but while she promotes the knowledge and skills of effective communication, her text, apart from occasional reference to issues of age, gender or language difference, proceeds as if these things are marginal concerns. Lishman presents an account of communication in which demographic differences are largely ignored or are overshadowed by an implicitly presumed, dominant white English culture. A culture in which, for the most part, language and meaning are personally constructed. The absence of sustained consideration of these issues seriously undermines the extent to which one can generalize from her precepts. Burnard (1989), in his advice to health professionals, similarly presents counselling as a set of skills and models divorced from consideration of the politics of language. Thus, apart from 'trying to avoid sexist language', there is little consideration of the role of language in constructing disadvantage, attitudes and identity. For the most part, language is presented as a neutral device.

While it might be pragmatic, indeed, to acknowledge the limits of social work, it is mistaken to assume that social work itself is not a political activity. As Dominelli (1988) has said, 'all social work is political, regardless of the perspective from which it is practised, because all social workers make decisions affecting other people's lives, and have the power to allow or deny people access to social resources. Social workers making these decisions within the parameters of the dominant ideology are not acting apolitically, they are reinforcing the status quo.' From an antidiscriminatory perspective, the absence of an account of how language reveals and constructs power is highly problematic.

As we shall see in the concluding chapter, the knowledge that we have of the role of language in building an antidiscriminatory practice is limited. This approach to practice is relatively new and, because it is overtly political, at both the personal and the social levels, it has the potential to create considerable professional and personal discomfort for us. Furthermore, acceptance of the approach requires the incorporation of much sociological and psychological knowledge which has not been fully established as part of the training and educational curriculum; therefore, it is important to recognize that in the development of this new paradigm for practice we are all, to some degree, novices.

7 Developing linguistically sensitive practice

> But if I had to speak English now, I'd never be able to say what's troubling me.
>
> *Translation of Welsh speaker, Davies, 1994*

INTRODUCTION

This chapter considers how we might begin to use knowledge about the complex relationship between language, thought, attitudes, identity and power within our work. This it attempts to do within the developing paradigm of antidiscriminatory practice.

Antidiscriminatory practice is not about selecting or choosing which 'ism' dominates or is most important: 'It is important to stress the importance of refusing to collude with the establishment of a hierarchy of more or less "worthy" oppression. Such a hierarchy allows those in power to pitch one set of political rights and demands against others' (Hudson, 1989). Rather, it is about recognizing that a person's situation in society, their life chances, power and problems are frequently determined by structural factors such as their membership of particular demographic groups. Membership is never confined to one category; an understanding of a person's situation has to encompass the multiplicity of potential determinants. For example, as Hugman (1991) recognizes, 'the experience and structural realities of black people differ between classes and between women and men'. However, at particular times and in specific circumstances, one or two of these factors may be most dominant in their consequences. For example, we should be aware that, unlike white non-English-speaking ethnic minorities, those whose first language is not English and who are also perceived as 'non-white' may find that the discrimination of racism is justified by reference to their lack of English (Baker, Husain and Saunders,

1991). It is through our knowledge of the probable consequences for particular groups that we are able to recognize the possible consequences for any individual member of these groups, though these, are not of course, inevitable.

A full review of what antidiscriminatory practice entails is beyond the scope of this book, but it should be apparent that it is not a 'bolt-on' or optional extra to existing theory and practice. Its use should not be restricted to situations when one is working with people who are identifiably different from oneself; it should be developed as an integral part of good practice *per se* (Davies, 1994; Dominelli, 1988; Thompson, 1993). It incorporates many of the key ideas traditionally associated with competent professional practice, namely, a clear value base, an explicit approach to the application of theory to practice, recognition of the primacy of the service user's needs and acceptance of the need to continually review theory and practice. The additional, distinctive features of antidiscriminatory practice arise from a broader sweep of analysis and from acceptance of the need to be proactive in our practice. For it is only from a thorough analysis of the needs and problems of service users, which incorporates at the micro level their culture, history and choices, and at the macro level an appreciation of the structural factors that can weigh so heavily upon their life chances and available options – that we are able to understand and effectively assist people. To do these things requires an understanding of the power that we possess and a willingness to use, share and sometimes disavow it.

Antidiscriminatory practice confronts all of us with knowledge about our more or less favoured locations in society. This is often discomforting to learn and, to the extent that it creates awareness of the possibility of conflict and confrontation with the interests and power of other people, may be unsettling to envisage. Nevertheless, while the starker forms of action may sometimes be necessary, careful assessment of intended action and probable consequence is vital, since thoughtless confrontation may be counterproductive. At the personal level, confrontation does not always bring illumination; instead it may create further barriers to understanding, while at the organizational level this effect may be magnified. Challenges to the power of people and organizations presents professionals with some of their most difficult dilemmas. In the most extreme situations, the experience of many whistle-blowers has shown the negative consequences of speaking out against inefficiency and injustice. However, not all of the changes required to institute antidiscriminatory practice lead inevitably to conflict, because many of the actions that create and reinforce discrimination are not intended to do so, but arise unwittingly from the implicit assumptions that underpin our thoughts and actions (Narayan, 1989). One consequence of this, as Ahmed has noted, is that 'the language barrier has been one of the most oppressive factors in denying many black and minority ethnic families their right to services, simply because the service agencies are not able to communicate with them in their own languages' (Ahmed, 1991).

RAISING OUR AWARENESS OF LANGUAGE

As noted in the discussion of Dominelli's work in the previous chapter, the first step in developing antidiscriminatory practice is to raise awareness of how discrimination operates and its effects. Within the antidiscriminatory perspective, there are three crucial elements which should form part of an enhanced awareness of language. It is important to recognize:

- **that there is no simple relationship between language and the external world**, that language both creates and sustains our ideas of what the world is like. Therefore, there is no universal objective external reality, but only our culturally learnt perceptions of our social world. Once this position has been understood, it is then possible to appreciate that other people's reality may be different from our own. Their reality is greatly, but not solely, determined by their social location and is reflected in the language that they use and the meaning attached to particular words and forms of language variation. For example, if a white, middle-aged, middle-class man used the word 'nigger' to describe a black person, the meaning would probably be intended, and understood, to be derogatory. However, the same word used by a young black man may not be understood in the same way: he might use it to reclaim the word and thus attempt to make its meaning positive rather than negative. He might use it consciously, as a knowing reference to his position in a racist society. Or he may have internalized the word and its negative meanings and thus, in repeating it, may unwittingly be sustaining its oppressive connotations.
- **that the choice of language as well as its content, carries meaning** – meaning about identity as well as intention and attitude. In the previous example, the word and who speaks it are the most significant forms of variation, which establish its meaning. But linguistic variation extends beyond vocabulary to differences in accent, dialect, code and type of language. For example, since Lithuania and the other Baltic states gained independence from the Soviet Union, Lithuanians who previously were forced to speak Russian at work and in dealings with officialdom now prefer to speak Lithuanian whenever possible. Latvian, the native language of the neighbouring state of Latvia, is similar to Lithuanian, but these two languages are not always mutually intelligible. Therefore, many Lithuanians, upon meeting a Latvian for the first time and in order not to be misidentified as Russian, will deliberately begin their conversation in Lithuanian before switching to Russian, which is also the second language spoken by most Latvians. This conscious switching of language not only facilitates communication, but also demonstrates a perception of commonality between the conversationalists, both perceiving each other and themselves as independent non-Russians.
- **that language and its expression reveals power and potentially creates and sustains it**. As a result, language is rarely neutral. It conveys particular

ideas about the world and expresses the nature of the relationship between the senders and the receivers of it. For example, in English the words 'her' and 'she' are often used to demonstrate possession or 'mastery' over inanimate things like boats. Whether the words are used by a man or a woman, they borrow from the social world the 'metaphorical gender' that we often use to categorize the world of non-human things. This categorization thus expresses our notions of dominance and subordination (Cameron, 1992). The relationship between language and power is complex and takes many forms. For example, it is worth noting that, although particular relationships or ideas may be conveyed by the use of specific words or languages, languages differ not only 'in what it is possible to say [but also in] what it is unavoidable to say' within them (Romaine, 1994). Such subtleties of meaning are frequently conveyed by the available forms of respectful address to other people. These are often highly structured. Within contemporary English-speaking societies such forms of personal address are not as formalized as in Japan or France, but nevertheless do exist and reveal significant information about power and status. For example, I saw a pre-sentence report that had been jointly written by two probation officers – a female officer had undertaken much of the initial research while a male colleague had written it up. At the end, his name was given, with the title 'Mr' followed by his initial and surname; her surname was rendered without a title, with her first name given in full! The male officer may have tried to avoid giving offence by not giving the woman a title that indicated her marital status. Unfortunately, he had not recognized that the use of a woman's first or given name often indicates an assumption of familiarity, let alone understood that the absence of any title at all could be seen as marking status difference.

Raising awareness should begin with an exploration of the attitudes to language held by individuals, those expressed by the practice of service organizations and those prevalent within the wider society. Attention should be focused in two directions: first to the majority language and especially to the unravelling of some of the implicit assumptions of superiority or naturalness and normality; second, to the attitudes held towards minority languages and those who speak them, as well as attitudes and assumptions about bilingualism. Davies, in a useful training pack aimed at increasing awareness of the Welsh language entitled *They All Speak English Anyway* (1994), has provided a series of exercises that assist this. Many of these exercises take the form of questions and statements that attempt to identify and clarify the reader's views on language. Most of these exercises are generic and can be used in any setting, and those that are specific to a Welsh context can usually be adapted to other situations.

WHAT KNOWLEDGE DO WE NEED?

Empirical knowledge about which languages are used and which are not within particular services and locations typically reveals mistaken assumptions about linguistic variation. The surprising range of diversity reported in the survey of London schools in Chapter 2 may not be representative of other locations, but there are few communities and services which do not contain some degree of linguistic variation. Health and welfare agencies should conduct research to establish the linguistic needs of their populations and, as well as identifying the range of linguistic variation, these should attempt to establish levels of communicative ability. This is a sensitive issue and self-rating questionnaires can be used to avoid the problem of externally imposed rating. Consultation with local ethnic minority groups and voluntary organizations can also provide valuable information and allay fears as to why such information is being sought. Following on from the basic awareness of linguistic and cultural variation, knowledge should be sought about personal and family naming systems, about respectful forms of address and about the systems of status and hierarchy used within different groups. A knowledge of the cultural rules of conversation shared within different groups should sensitize workers to the acceptable patterns and forms of question and response, and above all should avoid the unwitting giving of offence. This type of culturally specific information should also include knowledge of patterns of non-verbal communication and of important concepts such as time, health, illness and care (Leddy and Pepper, 1993).

Formal knowledge of the sociology, psychology and sociolinguistics of language, such as that reviewed in this book, should enhance awareness of the complexity of language use, and thus begin to make problematic the unthinking and taken-for-granted manner in which we often use language.

The following sections summarize some of the knowledge that is most useful when working in situations of linguistic, cultural and ethnic diversity.

ESTABLISHING COMMUNICATION

Davies (1994) cites the words of Anne Corsellis: 'Multilingualism isn't a problem, it's a fact. It only becomes a problem when you don't do anything about it.' This aptly summarizes the most important thing, which is the reality of language variation and our attitudes toward it. For many of us, the first shift that needs to take place is in our attitudes. We have to move to the perception that, when language difference exists, difficulty in communication is not the client's problem but **our** problem; both of us have a problem in understanding each other. Workers should always explicitly and respectfully acknowledge their own limitations with regard to knowledge of another person's language and culture. As Davis and Proctor (1989) have suggested, one of the first concerns that any prospective client has is the question, what does this person know about people like me? If the answer is effectively little or nothing, then there is no point in trying to disguise this fact, for it will soon become evident to the client. This acknowledgement and the expression of respect, together with a demonstrable willingness to learn and to check one's impressions, will help to establish credibility and goodwill, and so assist communication. White English monoglot workers often fail to appreciate how important respect is in other cultures; to fail to demonstrate it is a cause of shame, for it denies the 'face' of the other person. As Velasquez, Vigil and Benavides (1989) have pointed out in regard to Spanish speakers:

> In English one can respect another while violently opposing the opinions that that person holds. In English, respect does not contain the element of acceptance of another's view as one's own. *Respeto*, on the other hand, means that... if one chooses not to adopt the opinions of another as one's own, one must at least pay deference to the other person's views by not saying anything.
>
> *Velasquez, Vigil and Benavides, 1989*

Leaving aside for the moment the crucial questions of agency policy, statutory responsibility and any professional obligation to make services accessible, from the position of an English monoglot worker working within an agency where English is dominant, difficulties in communication because of language variation usually arise in one of the following four scenarios.

- The client understands little or no English and cannot speak it effectively at all.
- The client understands some English and speaks it a little.
- The client is bilingual, with English as the second language.
- The client is an English monoglot, but uses a different dialect, code or vocabulary from the service providers.

In the first case, there are two options for service providers – same-language provision or translation/interpretation. Same-language provision is the preferred option (refer also to the section on language policy), since the ready access provided by permanent employees who use the minority language as a matter of course will enhance accurate communication. There is a wealth of evidence that indicates how differences in client's cultural meanings, self-concept and patterns of communication impair effective therapeutic assessment (Marcos and Trujillo, 1981; Rack, 1982; Baptiste, 1984). For example, most Western health professionals, who come from cultures with high levels of verbal communication, become uncomfortable when faced with clients who pause often and are silent during communication. Frequently, they interrupt the silence, and usually have little idea of how to interpret its significance (Davidhizar and Giger, 1994). Berger and Luckman (1967) point out that the use of concepts like 'reality oriented' in psychiatric assessment are highly problematic if the psychiatrist is unaware of how much what we take for 'reality' is socially constructed, and hence socially variable. Thus, the culturally sensitive practitioner will, for example, 'arrive at different diagnoses of the individual who converses with the dead, depending upon whether such an individual comes from, say, New York City or from rural Haiti' (Berger and Luckman, 1967).

Translation and interpretation are terms which are sometimes used interchangeably, though technically their meanings differ. Translation usually refers to written text, while interpretation refers to spoken or signed languages. Unfortunately, as Ahmed has noted, 'in the absence of institutional acknowledgement and professional recognition of the role and status of interpreting, more often than not interpreting in minority community languages has remained cheap, ineffective and inadequate to the detriment of black and minority ethnic individuals and families in need of service' (Ahmed, 1991).

The most obvious 'technical' problem with translation and interpretation is that the conceptual framework of one language is often different from another. It is nearly always possible to find equivalent phrases and ideas, but this problem is more likely to occur when dealing with abstract subjects and is less likely to be picked up if the translator or interpreter is unaware of the possible slippage in meaning. Ideally, translators and interpreters should have experience in health and welfare services, so that they are familiar with the concepts and problems. However, the development of health and social work glossaries can assist in maintaining accuracy. Williams (1988b), for example, has provided a Welsh glossary of social work terminology, and Prys, Williams and Prys-Jones (1993) have provided a similar text on child care terminology. Translation of written material can be checked for accuracy by having another translator back-translate the text into the source language and then comparing it with the original. Other forms of establishing accuracy, such as testing the knowledge and performance of the recipient, are more onerous and carry obvious risks (Crystal, 1987).

When interpretation is required, it is important to understand the potential problems that derive from the use of another person to convey and elicit personal information.

Clients may be reluctant to provide sensitive information in the presence of a third person. Interpreters untrained in social work may impose their own meanings upon interaction. Alterations may arise unconsciously from differences between the perceptions and backgrounds of the interpreter and the client, for example, in caste or religion. Conscious alteration of content may occur when interpreters elicit information which they feel discredits their language group.

Pugh, 1992

Clearly, professional interpreters, trained in the relevant service and sensitive to the distinctions of meaning and the prevailing patterns of identity and social status within the language group, are generally to be preferred. However, the use of informal interpreters such as friends, neighbours and family members may on rare occasions have advantages as well as disadvantages. If the interpreter has been chosen by the client, it is more likely that they will feel comfortable expressing themselves through this other person. It is also likely that the interpreter will have a better grasp of the client's meanings. However, the client may be more reticent when they have no choice of interpreter, or when the information is sensitive or potentially embarrassing. In such instances, the neutrality of a professional interpreter may better facilitate disclosure. This is borne out by Baker, Husain and Saunders, (1991), whose research identifies a clear preference by service users for professional interpreters.

Except in cases of dire emergency, children should not be used to interpret for their parents or other adults. Not only may they be exposed to inappropriate information but they may be forced into a stressful role, in which they feel that they are totally responsible for their parents. Family roles may be further disrupted by the change in traditional patterns of communication and status. One important issue is, whose decision is it to use an interpreter? In my view, this should usually be the service user's, though sometimes, in working with children and people with mental health problems, the decision may legitimately be made by the worker. Usually, therefore, the choice should be offered to any prospective service user who speaks little or no English, or prefers to communicate through their own first language. Interpreters may also be necessary when both worker and a client share the same language, but are meeting with a third person who does not.

Mares, Henley and Baxter (1985) provide practical advice when using interpreters. They suggest that workers check that the client and the interpreter speak the same language and dialect, that the worker faces the client, not the interpreter, and that the interpreter must be briefed beforehand so that s/he is aware of the purpose of the meeting and of the point of particular questions. To this, I would add the importance of a debriefing afterwards, to allow feedback between the worker and the interpreter, and to allow additional clarification and feedback (Baker, Husain and Saunders, 1991). Mares, Henley and Baxter (1985) also make the crucial point that the interpreter is not an intermediary with regard to action and intervention; her/his purpose is solely to facilitate communication. Unfortunately, workers operating with clients from unfamiliar cultures have sometimes involved informal interpreters inappropriately, by asking them to take on tasks for which they are neither trained nor employed (Baker, Husain and Saunders, 1991).

In the second scenario, where the client understands some English and speaks it a little, the work of Mares, Henley and Baxter (1985) provides useful suggestions as to how communication may be enhanced. They propose that workers attempt the following:

- **to reduce the client's stress levels**. This can be done by allowing more time for the contact, giving appropriate reassurance and using appropriate non-verbal communication, using the person's name and pronouncing it correctly, using the same worker for all contacts with the client and always writing down the main points clearly for the client to take away with them.
- **to simplify the English used**. Workers should plan what they intend to say, identify the most significant points, avoid jargon and idiomatic English and

focus upon one thing at a time. They should speak slowly, repeating where necessary, initially using the same words in order to avoid confusion, but should not raise their voices and should always allow time for the client to absorb the information.

- **to seek feedback and keep checking**. This should be done frequently in order to avoid mounting confusion; the best feedback is to ask the client to explain what has been established or agreed, or is going to be done. Open questions are more likely to identify misunderstanding than closed ones: for example, 'Do you understand' is more likely to be met by a 'yes' than a 'no' from an anxious client.

It is in the third scenario, where the client is bilingual, with English as their second language, that some of the most thorny problems occur. As the discussion in Chapter 2 demonstrated, discriminatory attitudes towards minority languages, coupled with misconceptions about bilingualism, are legion. The assumption that a bilingual speaker has equal competence in each language and thus should be equally well served by a service delivered in either of their languages is mistaken. It assumes that the person's identity, attitudes, ideas and feelings are equally well represented in each; this is unlikely. Assuming that bilingual people have equal competence is likely to lead health professionals into thinking that the minority, non-English language is either irrelevant or 'merely a secondary problem – a nuisance factor – in having to deal with them' (Bellin, 1994). The integration of language and thought within people who are bilingual is complex. It is quite common for bilingual people to use one language and its associated thought patterns and meanings for one sphere of their life, and to use the second for others (Grosjean, 1982). This does not mean that bilingual people are linguistically schizophrenic but that they have an integrated approach to language, an approach and integration that is unique to each individual. The potential significance of this realization may be seen, for example, in child protection work, where a child may have learnt the names for body-parts in one language but may be used to dealing with adults from outside the immediate family in another. When relating distressing events, a bilingual person may prefer to use the language they feel most intimate in, but alternatively may prefer to use their second language because it may help to distance and dissociate them from the painful events.

Another problematic consequence that follows from the equal competence assumption is the tendency of people who are monoglots in the socially dominant language to assume that poor linguistic performance by bilingual people in this language is representative of their overall intellectual ability. Because there is no understanding of the way in which bilingual people learn and use language in different domains, and thus acquire different levels of competence according to the requirements of each domain, the general competence of the bilingual person is undervalued (Gumperz, 1982). In addition, there may be a further negative consequence, especially in situations where minority languages are devalued: because language is closely bound up with the construction of personal identity, bilingual people who speak the minority language may experience some degree of insecurity about the use of this language and/or themselves (Bellin, 1994). However, as the review of Tajfel's work in Chapter 3 indicated, reactions to perceived minority status are complex and cannot be accurately represented by simple dualities. The crucial point is that the provision of service in the language of the client's choice may avoid these problems or at least avoid exacerbating them.

In the fourth scenario, where the client is an English monoglot, but uses a different dialect, code or vocabulary from the service provider, there are a surprising number of possible pitfalls. Perhaps the most dangerous is when conversationalists assume that, because they speak the same language, they understand each other. In fact, there may be considerable drift between the comprehension of each. This type of problem may arise for different reasons. First, professionals may resort to language that obscures their meaning and intention. The phrase 'the double agenda' was coined to describe situations in which professionals and clients end up with different ideas about what is going on and what is going to happen next. Service providers can reduce the probability of this type of drift simply by being aware of its likelihood. Simple steps such as feedback, checking and summarizing are helpful. Health professionals should be aware that one factor which may explain their unwitting failure to communicate is their own impulse to self-protection. Satyamurti (1979) has noted how workers in stressful occupations, where they are uncertain and anxious or in situations where they are required to use authority, may use a number of symbolic means, including language, to distance themselves from the immediacy of events. 'The word "manipulative" is but one example of a range of linguistic and classificatory devices whereby social workers distanced their clients' (Satyamurti, 1979).

The second reason why drift occurs is because health professionals fail to understand how the meaning that a person attributes to events and expresses through language may vary according to a wide range of factors, not all of which are obvious to the unaware practitioner. Zulueta (1990) has noted how gender expectations are manifested within different languages in family therapy settings. In one case she describes a Colombian couple who both spoke English fluently. In English the husband presented 'as a fairly unassuming' man who seemed 'tolerant and gentle with his wife'. However, when observed speaking Spanish by a Spanish-speaking therapist, his language revealed a more powerful, 'macho' person who dominated his wife. Zulueta also notes that, where several languages are spoken within one family, the choice of language used can be a marker of power. In one French/Welsh/English-speaking family that were having problems, where the mother was first-language French and the father first-language Welsh, 'the mother used her children to maintain links with her French culture. The father could be seen to be redressing the balance of power by making his children learn his primary language at school. The linguistic difference highlights the marital split and the mother's social isolation.'

These examples are provided not to create the impression that bilingualism inevitably leads to problems, but to illustrate how workers who are unaware of such possibilities may unwittingly overlook the significance of the language choice exercised. The key is to recognize that language is not neutral, nor are its meanings universal and unchanging; it is not simply a tool of communication but is also the product and carrier of culture. Thus, as the discussion in the preceding chapters illustrates, context changes the meaning of words, non-verbal signs may contradict them, while power differences may inhibit the client's expression and response. The next section indicates some of the ways in which misunderstanding may be minimized.

CULTURALLY SENSITIVE ASSESSMENT

Boyle and Andrews (1989) have proposed an assessment model for nursing which attempts to avoid the problem of decontextualizing the patient's problem. They suggest eight aspects of the patient's background which should be considered; without undue oversimplification these can be summarized as:

- the social history of the cultural group;
- the ideas and value orientations toward such things as health, illness, ethics, social norms, magic, religion, law, time, money, work, change, food, education, politics, and so on;
- social and interpersonal relationship patterns and roles;
- patterns and forms of communication, and of consultation and decision making.

Clearly, this type of *pro forma* check or cultural grid framework (Pedersen and Pedersen, 1989) can be applied to virtually any of the welfare services; it basically seeks to avoid the omission of relevant material and prevent the fundamental error of 'cultural blindness' (Boyle and Andrews, 1989). A similar but more focused approach to elucidating the patient's cultural approach to illness has been proposed by Kleinman, Eisenerg and Good (1978). They suggest five basic questions to the patient.

- What do you think has caused your problem?
- Why do you think it started when it did?
- What do you think your illness does to you? How does it work?
- How severe is your sickness? Will it have a short or a long course?
- What kind of treatment do you think you should receive?

Both these approaches are likely to avoid the mistake of ethnocentrism, where the patient's experience is understood only from the perspective of the health professional and both are attempts to get at the patient's subjective perspective on her/his situation. For, as Zboroswki (1958) long ago demonstrated, even when different ethnic groups have similar responses to pain, the cultural meanings they attribute to their symptoms differ. Each of these approaches has some sensitivity to linguistic concerns, the first through explicitly asking about communication, and the second through avoiding the imposition of meaning.

Practitioners who are prepared to attempt to understand the meanings that people attach to their own words and behaviour are more likely to be able to reframe their initial perceptions of the other person into a more positive appreciation of their situation. After all, 'No one knows better the meaning of his [sic] own life, individual health status, and full circumstances integral to his own experiences than does the client himself. Thus, the client is the expert on the context' (Leddy and Pepper, 1993). Following the work of Harding and Hintikka (1983), Narayan (1989) has called this insider knowledge 'epistemic privilege', by which she means 'that members of an oppressed group have a more immediate, subtle and critical knowledge about the nature of their oppression than people who are non-members'. (This problem of 'centrality' is discussed further in Chapter 5.) This does not mean that non-members cannot develop an appreciation of the oppressed person's position, but that this appreciation is not easily achieved, nor will it always be complete, or directly felt. If we were to deny any possibility of appreciating the subjective reality of another person we could in effect deny the problem and evade any sense of responsibility for its amelioration. Acknowledgement of the epistemic privilege of insiders does not, however, imply that they necessarily 'have a clearer or better knowledge of the **causes** of their oppression' (Narayan, 1989). Thus, as we shall see later in this chapter, the disparity that arises when workers are better educated than their clients and perceive themselves to have better knowledge of the causes of their client's oppression can create powerful dilemmas in practice.

A rather different approach to checking the sensitivity of the assessment and subsequent intervention is to establish monitoring units within health and social service departments whose task is to offer advice and to review all service offered to ethnic minority service users. This has the advantage of concentrating expertise but, if insensitively implemented, can quickly lead to workers adopting defensive attitudes. Thus, cultural diversity becomes reinforced as a negative problem for workers. Such monitoring units, because they may be staffed by members from disadvantaged minorities, may result in a 'ghettoization' or marginalization of antidiscriminatory issues. Other staff may feel that, because there are 'experts', it is not necessary for them to take an interest or act; such a response is mistaken. The causes of discrimination do not arise from within the disadvantaged person or group but from the social responses of other people. For example, racism is exhibited towards those who are visibly different from the dominant white majority in Britain, but its cause is not the fact of black, brown or yellow skin, but lies in the attitudes and behaviour of white people to these differences. Because their responses are often based upon stereotypes and prejudicial opinions, logically the solution lies not with doing things to black, brown or yellow people, but in white people realizing that it is their own white attitudes and behaviour that are problematic (Dominelli, 1988; Ohri, 1982; Thompson, 1993).

THE NATURE OF THE RELATIONSHIP WITH SERVICE USERS

Recognition of power as an important variable in health and welfare practice has increased (Day, 1981; Hugman, 1991; Hawks, 1991; White, 1985, 1986, 1988; Walmsley *et al.*, 1993), and with this has come an acknowledgement of inequality. That is, an explicit acceptance of the fact that the health professional almost invariably stands in a position of superior power to the service user. Illich (1975) identified the potential of medical treatment to cause illness, and he called this process **iatrogenesis**. Awareness of iatrogenesis, that is of the potentially negative consequences of intervention, together with an awareness of inequalities of power, has stimulated a debate about the nature of the relationship with the service user (Brandon and Brandon, 1987; Brechin and Swain, 1987; Croft and Beresford, 1989). Under a variety of terms such as 'citizenship', 'consumerism', 'user involvement' and 'shared action planning', there has been a burgeoning interest in how health and welfare professionals relate to the public.

Empowerment has become the umbrella term used by many writers to encompass this new awareness and search for alternative forms of relationship and practice. 'Empowerment suggests that some people have power and have too much of it, other people have too little, and those who have too little should get more' (Gomm, 1993). However, as Gomm notes, this seemingly attractive concept is riven with ambiguity, meaning different things according to where people stand politically. Some of the practices described under the banner of empowerment, such as self-advocacy and groupwork, may clearly help users gain confidence and a voice, but these things do not in themselves necessarily alter the existing distribution of power. At the heart of many of the meanings is a strange paradox, which is that 'to empower someone else implies something that is granted by someone more powerful to someone who is less powerful: a gift of power, made from a position of power' (Gomm, 1993). I suggest that we should be more honest and accept that there is nearly always a fundamental inequality between service providers and service users, which derives not from the formal nature of the worker's employment, nor from the powers invested in them by law, though these factors are of course significant, but from the disparity in position between someone who seeks or is required to seek our services, and someone who does not (Compton and Galaway, 1989; Rojek, Peacock and Collins; 1988, Rodger, 1991). At the heart of the notion of empowerment is a recognition of this disparity and the premise that it should be minimized. For if there is no commitment to challenging oppressive practice then the concept remains merely a form of 'Newspeak [which] allows anyone to rewrite accounts of their practice without fundamentally changing the way it is experienced by service users' (Ward and Mullender, 1993).

By beginning with the client's perception of the problem we are able to appreciate her/his frame of reference and become consciously aware of how, whether and when we will introduce our perceptions of what is going on and what should happen. For example, a woman who has repeatedly been subjected to violence by her male partner may partly blame herself for precipitating his anger; her understanding of the problem is thus located primarily at the personal level and so she may not perceive any links between broader paternalistic assumptions about gender and her situation. This raises the tricky question about when, whether and how it is appropriate for a health professional to suggest that there are other ways of understanding the situation. Perhaps at the point when she is blaming herself, it would be appropriate for the worker not initially to provide a thoroughgoing feminist analysis of her situation, but to demur from her view of her own culpability and suggest that the responsibility for the violence is not hers but his. This may ease any sense of shame or guilt that she may feel about her predicament and pave the way to a different perception of this problematic relationship, its causes and the choices available to her. The worker may think that her/his perception of the woman's situation is the preferred and more accurate one, but change is unlikely unless the client, first, wishes to change and second, begins to reframe her experience in a different way. This reframing, however, should not be imposed by the worker, for as well as the questionable ethics of such imposition, it is unlikely to be successful unless the client is willing to accept the initial invitation to consider her situation differently. Either way, the worker's decision is inherently political in that the provision of information may begin to change the woman's perception of events and perhaps stimulate a change of action. Alternatively, by withholding it, the worker denies the client a potentially powerful source of information. All interaction is thus political, in the sense that it either enhances or reduces the possibilities for certain forms of thought and action.

The difficult task for workers is thus 'to acknowledge their power but not be paralysed into either inaction or authoritarianism by it' (Rodger, 1991). Most crucially, workers should avoid denying the power and the right of clients to speak for themselves. To deny this through the imposition of our supposedly superior knowledge and expertise not only increases the chances of misrepresentation of their experience but is likely to further diminish their 'sense of autonomy, identity and self-respect' (Narayan, 1989). In the absence of methods of working that allow clients and patients to participate and exercise some degree of agency, it is likely that the most effective way of them resisting the power of the professional is to remain silent and then refuse to comply by not following through with the recommended help/treatment. As Stimson and Webb (1993) have noted, 'while the patient's ability to control the outcome of the consultation is limited, he or she has considerable ability to control what happens after leaving the doctor's presence. In consultation the doctor makes the treatment decision; after the consultation, decision-making lies with the patient.'

EVALUATING PRACTICE

A thorough review of the evaluation of practice is beyond the scope of this book, but with regard to evaluation from an antidiscriminatory perspective it should be noted that at the present time there is little published material. It is possible that methods of evaluation which involve the service users are most likely to prove productive, but this is an area that requires further work (Pugh and Richards, 1996). This section is therefore fairly brief, but includes a useful self-assessment checklist and indications of where future development might profitably be focused.

Drawing heavily upon the ideas espoused by many counselling theorists, Hunsaker and Alessandra (1980) have developed a self-assessment checklist for evaluating one's own communication with other people. It is presented as a series of questions:

- Did I comprehend each point made?
- Did I make judgements of the words before the speaker was through speaking?
- Did I make decisions in my own mind while s/he was still speaking?
- Did I hunt for evidence that would prove the speaker right/wrong?
- Did I hunt for evidence that would prove myself right/wrong?
- Did I become upset while listening?
- Did I generally jump to conclusions while listening?
- Did I let the client speak at least 50% of the time?
- Did I understand the words in terms of their intended meanings?
- Did I restate ideas and feelings accurately?
- Did I study voice, posture, actions and facial expressions as the client talked?
- Did I listen between the lines for unspoken meanings behind the words?
- Did I really try to listen to the client?
- Did I really want to listen to the client?
- Did I really show the client I was, in fact, motivated and interested in listening to him [*sic*]? (Hunsaker and Alessandra, 1980)

Checklists like this are useful for sensitizing workers to these issues as well as for the intended purpose of evaluation. However, their obvious limitation is that they are self-administered. Consequently, it is relatively easy for workers to persuade themselves that they have operated positively. More useful results could be gained by asking other people to rate the effectiveness of the communication, either colleagues or clients. As the previous section indicated, because the most effective sanction that clients can exercise is to withdraw cooperation and compliance, problems in communication and in understanding of meaning are often only indicated by client silence. This may be one crude indicator of satisfaction.

Using client contact as an indicator may be inappropriate for some services. For example, in services where intervention is intentionally of short duration, such as advice shops, sexually transmitted disease clinics, X-ray and scanning departments, a return visit by the patient might be an indication of failure rather than success! Evaluation of the profile of service users is more easily undertaken and there is rather more experience in this field. The basic aim of such studies is usually to compare the actual profile of service users with the local populations from which they are drawn. Under- or over-representation of particular ethnic groups then becomes a focus for investigation. Examples of the results of this type of approach were described in Chapter 5. Another approach is to compare levels of service provision between similar agencies. Ideally the social composition of the two areas should also be similarly matched, but even if this is not possible, a crude comparison may raise important issues. For example, Baker, Husain and Saunders (1991) reported the findings of their survey of interpreters used by local authority social services departments and found that 39% of their respondents already employed full- or part-time interpreters, but that around 60% kept no records of their provision or the demand for the service.

Elsewhere, in other areas of service provision there are some disturbing conclusions. Ussher (1991), in her review of 'women's madness', identifies the misogynistic assumptions and stereotypes that have contributed to their over-representation as patients. Ussher attempts to untangle the web of causation and attribution, but does not deny the reality of the distress and experience of mental illness. Nevertheless, she clearly accepts the predominance of social factors when she approvingly cites Charlotte Perkins Gilmour, who wrote in 1892 'In a sick society, women who have difficulty fitting in are not ill but demonstrating a healthy positive response'. Ussher concludes that we should put aside our pet theories and listen directly to the experience of women. Similarly, the over-representation of black men in compulsory admissions for treatment and in their diagnosis also raises serious questions about society and professional practice (Rack, 1982; Littlewood and Lipsedge, 1982; Sashidharan, 1989). Not only are black patients diagnosed as 'schizophrenic' when the classic symptoms are absent, but new diagnoses have been created, such as 'ganja psychosis' and 'West Indian psychosis'. The powerful use of language to construct meaning is evident here: as Sashidharan states, these new categories not only pathologize the black community through the 'racialization of schizophrenia', but effectively articulate 'ideas about race – rather than about mental illness'. Similar studies have revealed disparities in the profiles of child care (Utting, 1991) and probation populations (Taylor, 1981). Cheetham's (1981) research for the Department of Health and Social Security has also shown the underuse of some of their services by black people. Thomas and Dines (1994), in a review of the nursing response to the health needs of ethnic minority groups, concluded that, while nurses accepted the principles of equality, their practice frequently failed to address real issues of communication, pain management and negative stereotyping. Most of the studies undertaken so far indicate that ethnic minorities are disadvantaged in two ways: first, they are over-represented in the 'corrective' areas of service and second, they are under-represented in the supportive areas of service. Access is often restricted by lack of information, ignorance of the needs of potential service users, language barriers and the ethnocentric assumption that all people's needs are the same.

There is a tendency in trying to assess antidiscriminatory practice to have an overbearing focus upon attitudes alone. This should be avoided, since it is by our actions and their consequences that our work is best judged. While it is tempting to spend a great deal of attention upon examining intentions, it can divert attention from consequences. Ward and Mullender (1993) warn of the dangers of superficially adopting the rhetoric of empowerment without really subscribing to its tenets. However, while I accept that the process of conscientization is frequently an uncomfortable one, I think their writing can be misread as overemphasizing the role of self reflection. By suggesting that a person should undergo 'the pain of confronting... [one's] own oppressive attitudes at a level deep enough to root them out', they are presenting an opportunity for the misuse of antidiscriminatory ideas and practice. Some so-called 'enlightened' practitioners may aggressively and oppressively seek to examine the attitudes of other less 'aware' practitioners. Ward and Mullender represent a rather static and one-sided view of the complex relationship between attitudes and behaviour. For if we recognize that good intentions may sometimes go awry in their implementation, we have to accept the possibility that superficially held and insufficiently understood ideas may sometimes also result in worthwhile outcomes. Furthermore, in the act of saying and doing, the less sophisticated but well-meaning practitioner may develop her/his appreciation of antidiscriminatory practice further. Apparently superficial compliance with antidiscriminatory principles may well be problematic, but it might be better evaluated by its consequences rather than by the depth of understanding. In the short term, the adherence to basic principles, whether cynically adopted or well-meant, can be irrelevant if the outcome for the client is satisfactory.

DEVELOPING LANGUAGE POLICY

Although most health and welfare agencies have equal opportunity policies which relate to aspects of disability, gender and 'race', very few have developed formal policies on language. For example, Baker, Husain and Saunders (1991), in a review of policies on interpreting within public services – which outlined the deleterious effects of language barriers upon service take-up and identified the *ad hoc* nature of many policies – argues that the right of ethnic minorities to participate equally in British society depends, in part, upon the provision of professional interpreters operating within clear guidelines and agreed policies. The absence of such policies means that both prospective employees and service users have little idea of what to expect from the service. With the exception of the Welsh Language Acts, successive governments have provided little or no leadership or statutory compulsion, so the needs of minority language groups are, for the most part, ignored. For example, while deaf people who use British Sign Language are the fourth largest language group in the UK, they are not recognized as a linguistic group by the Government or by most service providers. The predominantly rehabilitative approach to deafness ignores the fact that, for many deaf people, progress is limited and that this is an unsuccessful strategy which ignores deaf people's own acceptance and preference for signing. The imposition of the strategy of oralism and rehabilitation thus continues to define those who prefer to use sign language as having less than normal capacity, and so by implication they are perceived as abnormal (Taylor, 1993).

The National Health Service and Community Care Act 1990 makes no specific provision for language, although, in the assessment of care needs, workers are expected to consider the prospective service user in their social context. The principle of a needs-led assessment should encourage recognition of minority language. The 1983 Mental Health Act also omits any specific reference to language, though the latest Code of Practice does give guidelines for practice. Perhaps the most important of these is to consider the patient's cultural background when making an assessment for compulsory admission, and to interview the patient in a 'suitable manner'. This means that, where the patient and the health professional do not speak the same language, an interpreter should be used, ideally a professional one who also understands the cultural background of the patient. The guidance recommends that the authorities should make arrangements for a pool of interpreters and should advise doctors and approved social workers as to how they are to be used. However, as Davies (1994) has noted, the situation of bilingual patients who may understand the doctor or social worker's language but would prefer to speak in a 'minority' language such as Welsh is unclear.

Like these two Acts, the Children Act 1989 also promotes a client-centred approach to helping and protecting children. Thus in assessing a child's needs and making provision for them, the relevance of a child's cultural background is noted in Section 1, and the Act explicitly requires consideration of language in Sections 24, 64 and 74. However, even here there is potential ambiguity, since there is considerable scope for courts and social workers to interpret the requirement differently.

In Britain, in so far as the Government has a policy on language, it has moved from a form of language standardization (Nahir, 1977; Pugh, 1994b) to an element of language revival, or more accurately to a limited acknowledgement of linguistic variation in one of the four countries, that is, Wales. The 1967 Welsh Language Act, in principle, gave the Welsh language 'equal validity' with English in judicial matters and in the administration of government. Thus, Welsh could be used by witnesses and defendants in court in Wales, and Welsh language versions of government forms were made available. However, in practice the Act did little to promote access to health and welfare services. The 1993 Welsh Language Act goes further in requiring all public bodies to promote and facilitate the use of the Welsh language in their work. It also established a Welsh Language Board charged with the task of monitoring the Act's main provision, which is the requirement that all public bodies prepare and submit a language scheme that outlines their policy and plans for its implementation. The Act does not apply to private and independent organizations, nor does it confer the right to demand that a public service be delivered in Welsh. In the absence of real statutory 'teeth', the effectiveness of the Language Board will depend on how enthusiastically it pursues its brief, rather than upon its formal powers.

In the absence of clear statutory guidance on what a comprehensive language policy should contain, there are two useful sources from which to start – the work of CCETSW Cymru, the Welsh division of the Central Council for Education and Training in Social Work, and the Code of Practice for Interpreters outlined by Baker, Husain and Saunders (1991). The Code of Practice for Interpreters includes a statement of basic principles, advice on selection of interpreters and a process model for using and monitoring interpreting services. In Polisi yr Iaith Gymraeg/Welsh Language Policy (1989) and in their training pack *They All Speak English Anyway* (Davies, 1994) CCETSW Cymru have identified five core principles which they believe should guide practice.

- A client has the right to choose which language to use with a worker.
- Language is an essential part of a person's identity.
- A person can express feelings more effectively in a chosen language.
- Giving a client real choice regarding the use of language is the essence of good practice.
- Denying this right is a way of oppressing a client. (Davies, 1994)

CCETSW Cymru propose that these principles be clearly stated within an agency's policy documents, which should also contain practical strategies for the implementation of the policy, including guidelines for individual workers. This approach has obviously been developed to meet the perceived needs of social work clients and students within Wales, and explicitly recognizes the relationship of language to issues of identity and professional power. This policy and training pack provides a model of how other health and welfare agencies might begin to respond to their local needs.

The CCETSW Cymru approach is typical of what Mackey (1979) terms a 'personality' approach to language policy, that is, a policy which leaves the choice of language up to the individual person. It thus legitimates the person's right to choose but does not impose the actual choice. While this approach should promote the possibility of client choice by ensuring that service agencies are prepared to offer and respond to choice, it does have drawbacks. Most notably, it plays down the reality that many clients will not feel free to make their preferred choice unless they receive confirming evidence of the service's willingness and commitment to their language. In the absence of such evidence, all the other factors of attitude and power will come into play. As Williams

(1994), writing in a Welsh context, notes, 'When an agency refuses to share linguistic power, few are prepared to pay the price for insisting on a Welsh service.... It is better to receive some sort of service than no service at all; a client is unlikely to create further obstacles by refusing what is offered.' Consequently, in situations of relative powerlessness, clients will tend to adopt the language of the professional or adopt the one they perceive to have higher status (Pugh, 1992, 1994b). This is particularly likely to be the case with immigrants, who may wish to demonstrate that they are assimilating into the dominant culture. The underlying principle of the personality approach to language implies that all languages are equal, however 'the assumption of equal validity for minority languages is rather like the colour-blind [sic] approach to race, insofar as it assumes that all languages and people are equal at the point of intervention. They are not' (Pugh, 1994b).

An alternative approach to language is to establish a territorial policy (Mackey, 1979), which imposes the choice of language upon the client and the professional. Instead of the service accommodating to the individual, the individual has to accommodate to the language of the region or locale. This approach is used in Québec province in Canada and also in a number of European countries. In Switzerland, where there are four official languages, German, Italian, French and Romansch, each canton offers its services in the majority language of the district. For example, nationally French is a minority language spoken by only 18% of the total population, but in some cantons it is spoken by the majority and hence it is the territorially defined language.

Both types of policy have advantages and disadvantages; the naïve implementation of a personality policy, because it fails to see how choice is structured, is likely to further disadvantage the minority language speaker. Personality-based approaches are unlikely to succeed unless considerable effort is made to encourage and legitimize the client's possible choice. Bilingual signs, information and genuinely bilingual communication between staff will encourage people to feel that the choice offered is a real one without unfavourable consequences. The territorial approach avoids the problem of choice, but it is unlikely to succeed in areas where there is only a small proportion of minority language speakers. On a more limited local basis it might be a possible option. In terms of legitimating a minority group's choice of language, the establishment of offices and clinics operating monolingually in the preferred language would probably offer some of the benefits. However, where minority groups are already negatively stereotyped and subject to aggression and hostility, it may increase this by increasing their visibility. This is not a reason to avoid territoriality, since establishing the rights of minorities is often met with outright hostility by those who would deny them, but the negative possibilities should be borne in mind and planned for.

There is very little evaluative literature on policies for service delivery in areas of linguistic diversity. Most reports are more descriptive and either suggest that multilingual teams are the preferred means of response or propose linguistic specialization by some staff (Rack, 1982; Baptiste, 1984; Davis and Proctor, 1989). Specialization certainly facilitates communication, but it can be difficult to organize effective matching of client and worker and may also be counterproductive, as it tends to marginalize diversity instead of promoting acceptance of it as a normal part of service provision. While there has been relatively little research into language issues within health and social work, what there is indicates a need for training. Research into the effectiveness of counselling in situations of cultural difference suggests that ethnocentric curricula, together with a lack of appropriate training, are the main deficiencies (Arrendondo, 1985; Ponterotto and Casas, 1987; Sue and Sue, 1990). Taylor (1993) concludes that health professionals are poor at communicating with disabled people about sexual matters and suggests they need training in this area. From its own research, CCETSW Cymru has also recognized the need for greater awareness and training in language issues, though social service departments vary considerably in the extent to which they even perceive a problem, let alone react to it. Within the health service, the picture is similar: some training courses explicitly address language issues, but I suspect that many only superficially acknowledge language as a minor aspect of equal opportunity training.

Perhaps the most important aspect to be addressed in training is the frequent assumption that minority language use will eventually diminish as immigrants assimilate and the speakers of the older native tongues die out. While historically, most immigrants and their descendants have adopted English and languages like Gaelic have declined, we should be wary of assuming the inevitability of this process. The cultural resurgence of the Welsh language in television, radio, newspapers and popular music and public services has shown how unpredictable language revival can be. The increased interest and confidence in the language has confounded the pessimistic forecasts. We should also avoid presuming the desirability of minority language decline by implicitly assuming that there is one monoculture to which we will all eventually subscribe. As the discussion in Chapter 2 indicated, this is a nationalistic myth, albeit a powerful one.

CONCLUSION

Language is an important aspect of health and welfare practice that should not simply be subsumed under a general heading of race. It reflects the speaker's social history and social location in relation to that of the professional. Thus, an appreciation of the factors which shape language use is essential for the development of good practice. We have to accept that, in general, inequality in power between professional and client is an intrinsic problem which we may not solve, but might ameliorate through a conscious awareness of its untrammelled effects. The exploration and development of methods of intervention and policy formation which maximize the client's participation and capacity to make choices, is likely to ease some of these difficulties, though they will never be entirely absent.

An important step towards antidiscriminatory practice is to accept the reality of cultural and ethnic variation, to comprehend the cultural plurality that exists within our societies and to begin to view difference as a fact rather than a problem. With regard to minority languages and cultures, we should 'realize that the conceptual frames of reference they contain may have valuable lessons for mainstream culture (Fishman, 1988). They may embody concepts that remind us how the Western concepts of self and happiness are peculiarly individualistic and often separate from expectations of social role and obligation' (Pugh, 1994b). In developing language policies, we should take care to locate them within broader equal opportunity policies, so that implementation and evaluation are undertaken within a comprehensive antidiscriminatory perspective, a perspective that recognizes that each person is located on many different demographic dimensions, whose relative significance, in terms of our identity, the attitudes that others hold about us, and our power, varies.

Conclusion

The contention of this book is not that language alone should be the sole focus of analysis and theory, but that it is an essential element which is frequently ignored or underplayed. If we accept that language has a significant role in both creating and sustaining our social world and its meanings, then we should pay more attention to how it affects the everyday delivery of health and welfare. This book has focused upon the relationship between language, thought, attitudes, identity and power; it has attempted to review the knowledge that we have about how we use language and, in the accompanying chapters, to identify some of the more common problems within existing nursing and social work theory.

Most process models of nursing, social work and counselling, because they stress the importance of sensitivity, accurate communication, negotiation and feedback, have the potential to enhance culturally sensitive practice (Burnard, 1989; Compton and Galaway, 1989; Cournoyer, 1991). However, while they frequently recognize that it may be difficult to understand the subjective world of the client, they often implicitly 'assume that the meanings of language [itself] are fixed and definite' (Rodger, 1991). Additionally, their accounts of culture and society are typically rather static in their representations of social structure. Social features such as class and gender are often presented as being 'out there' somewhere, instead of being appreciated as social constructions created and represented through human interaction. As Giddens (1984), in his theory of structuration, has pointed out, the problem with analysing social structures as if they were really concrete and solid is that they become reified and human experience and opportunity are presented as being solely determined by birth, socialization and social location (Cassell, 1993). Consequently, the possibility of human agency or free will is negated by the pessimistic effects of an all-controlling determinism. At the heart of the problems in many health and welfare theories is an inadequate account of power: they fail to adequately recognize the extent to which we are both creative and created by our upbringing and experience and rarely recognize the crucial role of language in these processes.

Superficially, the discussion of the role of language within an antidiscriminatory perspective may have created the impression that it is solely an issue at the interpersonal level of communication. It is not. If we accept that language helps us to think and construct our internal ideas of the world and ourselves, then we have to recognize its unique position as the bridge between the internal and external worlds, between us and the others. The task for health and welfare professionals is therefore to develop forms of practice that are sensitive to the experience and understandings of our service users at the interpersonal level, while recognizing the impact of broader structural factors upon their experience and expectations of the service. Furthermore, we have to recognize that the prevailing discourses or paradigms within the human services are ones that have, historically, tended to underplay or omit recognition of the role that we play in reinforcing and representing existing forms of discrimination and disadvantage.

In an antiwelfare climate replete with the political rhetoric of low taxation and non-intervention, these are difficult times for health and welfare professionals as well as their service users; Taylor has concluded that

> whilst social workers are relatively powerful in relation to service users, they are increasingly powerless within their own organizations... which are themselves being made more accountable for their actions. The split between 'purchaser' and 'provider'... means... that the managers of care (the purchasers) are likely to have much higher professional status than the providers of care, but within a much more administrative regime.
>
> *Taylor, 1993*

This statement could apply to virtually any branch of health and welfare for it sums up the present difficulties with regard to the diminution of professional power. Arguably, this diminution could be welcomed if it heralded a redistribution from the professional to the service user, but it does not; the apparently inexorable centralization of power in modern states continues unabated. In the meantime, within the opportunities that are afforded us, we must continue to refine our practice at the micro level of interaction with clients and should accept the political necessity of advocacy on behalf of those service users whose voice is not heard, or future users whose needs have not yet become apparent. This situation has parallels with the situation in the late 19th and early 20th century, when social researchers and activists not only collected information to demonstrate the extent of need but effectively challenged the prevailing paradigm about what was possible. In the post-modern era, where fragmentation and the retreat from rationality are all too easily conceded, we should remember that the Victorians, once dubbed the 'reluctant collectivists', eventually accepted the necessity of wholesale intervention, in part because the market could not or would not provide for society's weakest members and in part from fears of social unrest. Such unrest is built upon a platform of perception and information; the question facing health and welfare professionals today is to decide whether it is our role to provide this.

Glossary

Ageism: Discriminatory attitudes, behaviour and social structures that disadvantage people on the basis of their age.

Communication: The transmission of information, by speech, movement, gesture, expression, writing, sign or other symbol, from one person to another.

Communicative competence: The ability, consciously or unconsciously, to use language appropriately in different social situations. It encompasses the explicit and tacit 'rules' that guide the interaction and allow meaning to be inferred and attributed to utterances.

Constructionism: A theoretical approach to the study of human psychology and society which proposes that there is no universal human reality but that society, cultures, groups and individuals each build or create their own version of what is perceived as reality. Thus things seem and are real to people because they are the usual or normal ways of thinking about things within their cultural group.

Conversation analysis: The study of actual conversations between people and the identification of the implicit rules that govern them.

Culture: The common features of custom, belief, values and ideas embodied and expressed through the language and behaviour of particular social groups. *See also* Ethnicity.

Deconstructionism: A form of analysis that attempts to demonstrate the socially constructed nature of an idea or text. It tries to show how ideas are 'of their time' and rejects the notion of absolute truth. Usually it is done by close analysis of the words and ideas contained within a text and not only seeks to indicate their origin but points out alternative ideas that have been avoided or insufficiently explored.

Demography: The study of populations and their size and composition. Hence the term demographic factor typically refers to dimensions of difference such as age, sex and ethnicity.

Determinism: The view that all human action is determined by external causes;

typically this approach attributes causation to a single factor such as social class, human genes and so on. This stance can be criticized for denying any capacity for agency (free will) and for failing to reflect the complex and multiple factors that influence human behaviour.

Discrimination: Behaviour that disadvantages individuals and social groups from sharing in or achieving the rewards and opportunities available to others.

Discourse: This notion comes originally from linguistics, where it refers to a piece of text or conversation, but it has developed a broader meaning: it is a recognition that words and language are not neutral entities separated from the socially constructed realities we live in, but are part of them. Thus they inevitably represent, directly or indirectly, particular ideas about ourselves and our social worlds, and those of other people. Discourse analysis also seeks to identify what is unsaid, in the sense that a discourse excludes other ways of looking at situations. *See also* Constructionism, Deconstructionism.

Empiricism: The philosophical belief that knowledge can only be developed through the direct observation or acquisition of data or facts. In this text the term **empirical** is used, in a less precise way, to refer to any activity in which direct contact is made with the object/subject of study, as opposed to more distanced, abstract theoretical speculation.

Epistemology: Epistemologies are theories of knowledge that analyse the nature of the relationship between the thinker and the subject of her/his thought. Epistemology thus seeks to answer a fundamental question: how is it we know something and what is the status of such knowledge? Therefore, epistemological questions are concerned with truth and whether it exists, with whether we can really appreciate the subjective experience of another person, and so on.

Ethnicity: The common features of behaviour, ideas, language, values and meaning that are held by members of social groups who share and have a subjective awareness of common identity. These common features may also include diet, dress, religion and physical appearance, including such things as skin colour. Ethnicity is to a large degree situational, in that both the extent of cultural distinctiveness and the particular ethnic features that a group is identified by vary according to social circumstances.

Ethnocentrism: The appreciation, interpretation and understanding of other cultures through the perspective of one's own culture. This leads to misunderstanding and misreading of meaning and significance and also the tendency to derogate that which is different.

Ethnomethodology: The study of society from the perspective of the various groups that comprise it. This is an appreciative approach that attempts to understand the subjective realities held by different people and to identify the common-sense, taken-for-granted aspects of everyday life.

Gender: The socially learned ideas and roles attributed to male and female biological difference; hence, stereotypical ideas of femininity and masculinity.

Ideology: This is a contested concept, but it is often used to refer to particular ideas, beliefs and ways of seeing the world that legitimate existing social arrangement. In its pejorative connotation it suggests false and irrational notions. Thus, while an ideology may be widely held by many people, the overall effect is to justify the advantageous and relatively powerful position of the most dominant group.

Linguist: The conventional use of this word refers to someone who learns about a language or speaks several languages. The technical use of the term within linguistics means someone who studies languages in a scientific or academic manner. The terms **linguistic theorist** and **linguistician** were previously used to signal this distinction, but latterly **linguist** has become the preferred term.

Minority group: People who are in a disadvantaged position in society because of some physical, cultural, ethnic or other social difference from the dominant group. The term **minority** refers more to relative power and opportunity than to relative groups size; thus women, though numerically dominant, are in most paternalistic societies nevertheless treated as a second-rate group.

Nationalism: The concept of the large social group which self-identifies as a nation is associated with a particular homeland or territory. Nationalism is conveyed by beliefs and ideology and is represented through symbols such as flags and languages.

Paradigm: Originally this referred to the notion that in science there was at any given time a prevailing world view about the natural world and the 'laws' that regulate or explain it. Paradigms are the accepted conventional wisdom that is adhered to and accepted by the scientific establishment. Changes or shifts in paradigms do occur, but are often resisted by those who accept the prevailing world view. Thus Galileo, Newton and Einstein have each stimulated a paradigm shift with their work. The notion of paradigm has been imported into the social sciences and is similar to the idea of discourse, except that, where a discourse may be unconsciously represented, the supporters of a paradigm are usually fully aware of their position.

Power: Another highly contested concept, but frequently used to refer to the capacity of people or groups to achieve their desired aims through the manipulation of their social and physical environment.

Prejudice: The preconceived, pre-existing and thus prejudged ideas held about particular people and groups, which remain unchanged even when challenged by new or contradictory information.

Racism: This is a specialized form of discrimination in which there is a mistaken presumption that there are separate and different human races. These are believed to be identifiable by their specific physical or social characteristics, and the core of the belief is the notion that some races are inherently superior while others are inherently inferior. In this way racism is a form of ideology because it is used to justify the unfavourable treatment of one group to the benefit of others. Racism operates at the personal, the cultural and the institutional levels of society, so that its effects are manifested throughout the ideas, behaviour and structures of a society.

Reductionism: Any attempt to reduce a phenomenon to the basic elements that are believed to constitute it; this approach is widely used in the natural sciences, where it is possible to identify the constituent chemical elements of many substances. However, within the social sciences the approach may lead to oversimplification of complex phenomena and failure to appreciate the significance or meaning of behaviour that may only be comprehended 'in the whole'.

Reification: To treat an abstract idea or concept as if it were actually a concrete entity. This is not to deny the importance of the beliefs that people have in, say, God or social class, but to recognize that the reality of these concepts is constructed within people's minds and by their behaviour rather than existing as concrete structures separated from human cognition.

Role: The idea that people learn and act the behaviour that is expected in certain situations or positions.

Semiotics: The study of signs, their use and their meaning.

Sexism: A specialized form of discrimination based upon a belief in the innate superiority of men over women. In less obvious forms, it can be identified by ideas and actions that, while not overtly intending to disadvantage women, nevertheless do so. Like racism, it operates from the personal to the institutional levels of society and is replicated through the attitudes and behaviour of individuals and the organizational practices of employers and public bodies.

Sexuality: The sexual behaviour and preference of a person or group.

Social structure: Usually taken to refer to the invisible but stable aspects of a society represented by such concepts as social class and gender. Frequently, these are assumed to be solid and fixed structures as if they had physical qualities but, following the work of writers like Berger and Luckman (1966) and Giddens (1984) they are now seen not to exist outside of people but to be created and re-created through their actions, the meanings they attribute to them and the effects upon other people. *See also* **Deconstructionism**.

Stereotype: A simplified conceptual category or picture of a person, group or thing which either misrepresents particular features or exaggerates them, Stereotypes may be positive or negative in the perceptions they present.

Symbol: An object, sound or sign that represents or stands for some other meaning or thing.

References

Aaron, J., Rees, T., Betts, S. and Vincentelli, M. eds (1994) *Our Sisters' Land: The Changing Identities of Women in Wales,* University of Wales Press, Cardiff.

Ahmed, B. (1991) Preface, in *Interpreters in Public Services,* (eds Baker, P., Hussain, Z. and Saunders, J.), Venture Press, Birmingham.

Ahmed, S. (1978) Asian girls and cultural conflicts. *Social Work Today*, August.

Ajzen, I. (1988) *Attitudes, Personality and Behaviour*, Open University Press, Milton Keynes.

Akinasso, F.N. (1982) On the differences between spoken and written languages. *Language and Speech,* 25, 97–125.

Ali, D., Momen, R. and Bhuia, J. (1995) *Who Cares For Us?*, Social Services Strategy Group, Tower Hamlets, London.

Alladina, S. and Edwards, V. (1991) *Multilingualism in the British Isles,* vols 1 and 2, Longman, Harlow.

Althusser, L. (1971) *Lenin and Philosophy and Other Essays*, New Left Books, London.

Anderson, B. (1983) *Imagined Communities: Reflections on the Origin and Spread of Nationalism*, New Left Books, London.

Argyle, M. (1975) *Bodily Communication*, Methuen, London.

Argyle, M. (1983) *The Psychology of Interpersonal Behaviour*, Penguin, Harmondsworth.

Arrendondo, P. (1985) Cross-cultural counselor education and training, in *Handbook of Cross-Cultural Counseling and Therapy*, (ed. P.B. Pedersen), Greenwood Press, Westport, CT.

Atkinson, P. (1988) Ethnomethodology: A critical review. *Annual Review of Sociology*, 14, 441–465.

Ayto, J. (1993) *Euphemisms*, Bloomsbury Press, London.

Baker, C. (1992) *Attitudes and Language*, Multilingual Matters, Clevedon, Avon.

Baker, C., Arseneault, A.M. and Gallant, G. (1994) Resettlement without the support of an ethnocultural community. *Journal of Advanced Nursing*, 20, 1064–1072.

Baker, P., Husain, Z. and Saunders J. (1991) *Interpreters in Public Services*, Venture Press, Birmingham.

Bakewell, D. (1992) Publish in English, or perish. *Nature*, 356, 648.

Bamford, T. (1990) *The Future of Social Work*, Macmillan, London.

Baptiste, D.A. (1984) Marital and family therapy with racially/culturally intermarried step-families: Issues and guidelines. *Family Relations*, 33, 373–380.

Barrett, E.A.M. (1989) A nursing theory of power for nursing practice: Derivation from Roger's paradigm, in *Conceptual Models for Nursing Practice*, (ed. J. Riehl-Sisca), Appleton & Lange, East Norwalk, CT, pp. 207–217.

Baugh, A.C. and Cable, T. (1993) *A History of the English Language*, Routledge, London.

Becker, H.S. (1963) *Outsiders: Studies in the Sociology of Deviance*, Free Press, New York.

Bellin, W. (1994) Caring professions and Welsh speakers: A perspective from language and social psychology. *Gwaith Cymdeithasol a'r Iaith Gymraeg/Social Work and The Welsh Language*, (eds R.H. Williams, H. Williams and E. Davis), University of Wales Press, Cardiff, pp. 75–121.

Benner, P. (1985) Quality of life: A phenomenological perspective on explanation, prediction and understanding in nursing science. *Advanced Nursing Science*, 8, 1–14.

Berger, C.R. and Calabrese, R.J. (1975) Some explorations in initial interaction and beyond: Towards a developmental theory of interpersonal communication. *Human Communication Research*, 1, 99–112.

Berger, P.L. and Luckman, T. (1967) *The Social Construction of Reality*, Penguin, Harmondsworth.

Berlo, D.K. (1960) *The Process of Communication*, Holt, Rinehart & Winston, New York.

Berne, E. (1968) *Games People Play*, Penguin, Harmondsworth.

Bernstein, B. (1973) *Class, Codes and Control*, Routledge & Kegan Paul, London.

Bilingual Education Act 1968 *PL 90-247, Title vii, 81 Stat. 816*, Washington, DC.

Billig, M. (1976) *Social Psychology and Intergroup Relations*, Academic Press, London.

Black, M. and Coward, R. (1990) Linguistic, social and sexual relations: A review of Dale Spender's *Man Made Language*, in *The Feminist Critique of Language: A Reader*, (ed. D. Cameron), Routledge, London.

Blattner, B. (1981) *Holistic Nursing Care*, Prentice Hall, New York.

Bloomfield, L. (1933) *Language*, Holt, Rinehart & Winston, New York.

Bor, R., Perry, L. and Miller, R. (1993) When the solution becomes part of the problem, in *Health, Welfare and Practice*, (eds J. Walmsley, J. Reynolds, P. Shakespeare and R. Woolfe), Sage Publications, London, pp. 227–230.

Borland, J., Fevre, R. and Denney, D. (1992) Nationalism and community in North Wales, in *Sociological Review*, 40, 49–72.

Bourhis, R.Y. (1984) Language policies in multilingual settings, in *Conflict and Language Planning in Quebec*, (ed. R.Y. Bourhis), Multilingual Matters, Clevedon, pp. 1–28.

Boyle, C.M. (1975) Differences between patients' and doctors' interpretations of some common medical terms, in *A Sociology of Medical Practice*, (eds C. Cox and A. Meads), Collier-Macmillan, London.

Boyle, J.S. and Andrews, M.M. (1989) *Transcultural Concepts in Nursing Care*, Scott, Foresman/Little, Brown College Division, Glenview, IL.

Brandon, A. and Brandon, D. (1987) *Consumers as Colleagues*, MIND, London.

Brazil, D., Coulthard, M. and Johns, C. (1980) *Discourse Intonation and Language Teaching*, Longman, London.

Brechin, A. and Swain, J. (1987) *Changing Relationships – Shared Action Planning for People With Mental Handicaps*, Harper & Row, London.

Brown, B.L. (1980) Effects of speech rates on personality attributions and competency evaluations, in *Language: Social Psychological Perspectives,* (eds H. Giles, W.P. Robinson and P. Smith), Pergamon, Oxford, pp. 294–300.

Brown, B.L., Giles, H. and Thackerar, J.N. (1985) Speaker evaluations as a function of speech rate, accent and context. *Language and Communications,* 5, 207–220.

Bruni, N. (1989) Holism: A radical nursing perspective, in *Theory and Practice: An Evolving Perspective*, (ed. T. Koch), School of Nursing Studies, Sturt, South Australia.

Bryson, B. (1990) *Mother Tongue: The English Language*, Penguin, Harmondsworth.

Burgoon, M., Birk, T.S. and Hall, J.R. (1991) Compliance and satisfaction with physician–patient communication: An expectancy theory interpretation of gender differences. *Human Communication Research*, 18, 177–208.

Burgoon, B., Hunsaker, F.G. and Dawson, E.J. (1994) *Human Communication*, Sage Publications, London.Burgoon, B., Hunsaker, F. G. and Dawson, E. J. (1994) *Human Communication*, Sage Publications, London.

Burgoon, M., Jones, S.B. and Stewart, D. (1975) Toward a message-centered theory of persuasion: Three empirical investigations of language intensity. *Human Communication Research*, 1, 240–256.

Burkitt, I. (1991) *Social Selves: Theories of the Social Formation of Personality*, Sage Publications, London.

Burnard, P. (1989) *Counselling Skills for Health Professionals*, Chapman & Hall, London.

Caine, N. (1993) Summer romances, lifetime promises. *The Independent*, 7 October, p. 22.

Cameron, D. (ed.) (1990) *The Feminist Critique of Language: A Reader*, Routledge, London.

Cameron, D. (1992) *Feminism and Linguistic Theory*, Macmillan, London.

Campbell, B. (1994) A personal urge to control. *The Independent*, 26 October, p. 15.

Carter, H. and Aitchison, J. (1986) Language areas and language change in Wales: 1961–1981, in *The Welsh and their Country*, (eds I. Hume and W.T.R. Pryce), Gomer, Llandysul, Dyfed, pp. 1–25.

Cashmore, E. and Troyna, B. (1982) *Black Youth in Crisis*, Allen & Unwin, London.

Cashmore, E. and Troyna, B. (1983) *An Introduction to Race Relations*, Routledge & Kegan Paul, London.

Cassell, P. (1993) *The Giddens Reader*, Macmillan, London.

Castex, G.M. (1994) Providing services to Hispanic/Latino populations: Profiles in diversity. *Social Work: Journal of the National Association of Social Workers*, 39, 288–296.

CCETSW (1989) *Welsh Language Policy/Polisi yr Iaith Gymraeg*, CCETSW, Cardiff.

Chapman, G. (1993) Rituals and rational action in hospitals, in *Health, Welfare and Practice: Reflecting on Roles and Relationships*, (eds J. Walmsley, J. Reynolds, P. Shakespeare and R. Woolfe), Sage Publications, London, pp. 190–195.

Cheetham, J. (1981) *Social Work Services for Ethnic Minorities in Britain and the USA*, DHSS, London.

Children Act 1989, HMSO, London

Chinn, P.L. and Kramer, M.K. (1991) *Theory and Nursing: A Systematic Approach*, Mosby-Year Book, Philadelphia, PA.

Chomsky, N. (1968) *Language and Thought*, Harcourt Brace, New York.

Chomsky, N. (1986) *Knowledge of Language: Its Nature, Origins and Use*, Praeger, New York.

Cicourel, A. (1973) *Cognitive Sociology*, Penguin, Harmondsworth.

Clarke, J. (ed.) (1993) *A Crisis in Care; Challenges to Social Work*, Sage Publications, London.

Classen, C. (1993) *Worlds of Sense: Exploring the Senses in History and Culture*, Routledge, London.

Coates, D. (1984) *The Context of British Politics*, Hutchinson, London.

Coates, J. (1993) *Women, Men and Language*, Longman, Harlow.

Code of Practice to the Mental Health Act 1983 (1990) HMSO, London.

Cole, M and Cole, S. (eds) (1979) *The Making of Mind: A Personal Account of Soviet Psychology, Alexander Romanovich Luria (1902–1977)*, Harvard University Press, Cambridge, MA.

Compton, B.R. and Galaway, B. (1989) *Social Work Processes*, Brooks Cole, Pacific Grove, CA.

Coupland, N. and Giles, H. (1988) Introduction: The communicative contexts of accommodation. *Language and Communication*, 8, 175–182.

Cournoyer, B. (1991) *The Social Work Skills Handbook*, Wadsworth, Belmont, CA.

Croft, S. and Beresford, P. (1989) User involvement, citizenship and social policy. *Critical Social Policy*, 26, 5–18.

Cross, W.E. (1971) The Negro to Black conversion experience: Towards a psychology of Black Liberation, *Black World*, 20, 13–27.

Cross, W.E. (1978) Models of psychological Nigrosence: A literature review, *Journal of Black Psychology*, 5, 13–31.

Crow Dog, M. and Erdoes, R. (1991) *Lakota Woman*, Harper Collins, New York.

Crystal, D. (1987) *The Cambridge Encyclopedia of Language*, Cambridge University Press, Cambridge.

Czechmeister, C.A. (1994) Metaphor in illness and nursing: A two-edged sword. A discussion of the social use of metaphor in everyday language, and implications of nursing and nursing research. *Journal of Advanced Nursing*, 19, 1226–1233.

Dahrendorf, R. (1973) *Homo Sociologicus*, Routledge & Kegan Paul, London.

Dallos, R. and Sapsford, R.J. (1981) The person and group reality, in *Crime and Society: Readings in History and Theory*, (eds M Fitzgerald, G. McLennan and J. Pawson), Routledge & Kegan Paul, London, pp. 429–459.

Davidhizar, R. and Giger, N.J. (1994) When your patient is silent. *Journal of Advanced Nursing*, 20, 703–706.

Davies, E. (1994) *They All Speak English Anyway*, CCETSW Cymru, Cardiff.

Davies, L.E. and Proctor, E.K. (1989) *Race, Gender and Class: Guidelines for Practice with Individuals, Families and Groups*, Prentice Hall, Englewood Cliffs, NJ.

Davies, M. (1985) *The Essential Social Worker: A Guide to Positive Practice*, Gower, Aldershot.

Davis, K. (1991) Critical sociology and gender relations, in *The Gender of Power*, (eds K. Davis, M. Leijenaar and J. Oldersma), Sage Publications, London, pp. 65–86.

Day, P.R. (1981) *Social Work and Social Control*, Tavistock, London.

Deising, P. (1971) *Patterns of Discovery in the Social Sciences*, Aldine-Atherton, Chicago, IL.

Department of Education and Science and Welsh Office (1988) *English for Ages 5–11: Proposals of the Secretary of State for Education and Science and the Secretary of State for Wales*, HMSO, London.

Derrida, J. (1987) *The Post-Card: From Socrates to Freud and Beyond*, University of Chicago Press, Chicago, IL.

Dobson, C.B., Hardy, M., Heyes, S. *et al.* (1982) *Understanding Psychology*, Weidenfeld & Nicolson, London.

Dominelli, L. (1988) *Anti Racist Social Work*, Macmillan, London.

Durkheim, E. (1938) *The Rules of Sociological Method,* Free Press, New York.

Edwards, G. (1992) *Sociolinguistics: A Sociological Critique*, Routledge, London.

Edwards, J. (1994) *Multilingualism*, Routledge, London.

Edwards, J.R. (1977) Ethnic identity and bilingual education. *European Monographs in Social Psychology*, 13, 250–269.

Edwards, V. (1986) *Language in a Black Community*, Multilingual Matters, Clevedon, Avon.

Ellis, A. and Beattie, G. (1986) *The Psychology of Language and Communication*, LEA, Hove, East Sussex.

Ely, P. and Denney, D. (1987) *Social Work in a Multi-Racial Society*, Gower, Aldershot.

Ervin-Tripp, S. (1972) Sociolinguistic rules of address, in *Sociolinguistics*, (eds J.B. Pride and J. Holmes), Penguin, Harmondsworth, pp. 225–240.

Ervin-Tripp, S. and Gordon, D. (1986) The development of requests, in *Language Competence: Acquisition and Intervention,* (ed. R.L. Schiefelbusch), Taylor & Francis, London, pp. 61–95.

Finkelstein, V. and French, S. (1993) Towards a psychology of disability, in *Disabling Barriers – Enabling Environments*, (eds J. Swain, V. Finkelstein, S. French and M. Oliver), Sage Publications, London, pp. 2633.

Fishman, J.A. (1972) The relationship between micro- and macro-sociolinguistics in the study of who speaks what language to whom and when, in *Sociolinguistics*, (eds J.B. Pride and J. Holmes), Penguin, Harmondsworth, pp. 15–32.

Fishman, J.A. (1977) Language and ethnicity. *European Monographs in Social Psychology*, 13, 15–36.

Fishman, J.A. (1980) The Whorfian hypothesis: Varieties of valuation, confirmation and disconfirmation. *International Journal of the Sociology of Language,* 26, 25–41.

Fishman, J.A. (1988) *Language and Ethnicity in Minority Sociolinguistic Perspective*, Multilingual Matters, Clevedon, Avon.

Fishman, P.M. (1978) Interaction: The work women do. *Social Problems*, 24, 397–406.

Flynn, P.A.R. (1980) *Holistic Health*, Robert J. Brady, Bowie, MD.

Forder, A. (1976) Social work and systems theory. *British Journal of Social Work*, 6, 24–41.

Foucault, M. (1967) *Madness and Civilisation: A History of Insanity*, Tavistock, London.

Foucault, M. (1972) *The Archeology of Knowledge*, Tavistock, London.

Foucault, M. (1977) *Discipline and Punish: The Birth of the Prison*, Allen Lane, London.

Foucault, M. (1979) *The History of Sexuality, Volume 1: An Introduction*, Allen Lane, London.

Foucault, M. (1988) Technologies of the self, in *Technologies of the Self* (eds. L.H. Martin, H. Gutman and P.H. Hutton), Tavistock, London.

Fowler, R., Hodge, B., Kress, G and Trew, T. (1979) *Language and Control*, Routledge & Kegan Paul, London.

Fraser, B. (1980) Conversational mitigation. *Journal of Pragmatics*, 4, 341–350.

Freund, J. (1968) *The Sociology of Max Weber*, (trans. M. Ilford), Penguin, Harmondsworth.

Gal, S. (1979) *Language Shift: Social Determinants of Linguistic Change in Bilingual Austria*, Academic Press, New York.

Garfinkel, H. (1967) *Studies in Ethnomethodology*, Prentice Hall, Englewood Cliffs, NJ.

George, N. (1994) Blackface: Reflections on African-Americans and the movies, cited in S. O'Hagan, Georgian ethics. *The Guardian*, 3 September.

George, V. and Wilding, P. (1976) *Ideology and Social Welfare*, Routledge & Kegan Paul, London.

Giddens, A. (1976) *New Rules of Sociological Method*, Hutchinson, London.

Giddens, A. (1984) *The Constitution of Society*, Polity Press, Cambridge.

Giddens, A. (1991) *Modernity and Self Identity: Self and Society in the Late Modern Age,* Stanford University Press, San Francisco, CA.

Giles, H., Bourhis, R.Y. and Taylor, D.M. (1977) Towards a theory of language in ethnic group relations. *European Monographs in Social Psychology*, 13, 310–331.

Goffman, E. (1959) *The Presentation of Self in Everyday Life*, Doubleday, New York.

Goffman, E. (1961) *Asylums: Essays on the Social Situation of Mental Patients and Other Inmates,* Doubleday Anchor, New York.

Goffman, E. (1968) *Stigma: Notes on the Management of Spoiled Identity*, Pelican, Harmondsworth.

Goffman, E. (1974) *Frame Analysis*, Harper, New York.

Goldman, L. (1964) *The Hidden God*, Routledge & Kegan Paul, London.

Goldstein, H. (1973) *Social Work Practice: A Unitary Approach*, University of South Carolina Press, Columbia, SC.

Gomm, R. (1993) Issues of power in health and welfare, in *Health, Welfare and Practice*, (eds J. Walmsley, J. Reynolds, P. Shakespeare and R. Woolfe), Sage Publications, London, pp. 131–137.

Gramsci, A. (1971) *Selections from the Prison Notebooks*, Lawrence & Wishart, London.

Greene, J. (1975) *Thinking and Language,* Methuen, London.

Grosjean, F. (1982) *Life with Two Languages*, Harvard University Press, Cambridge, MA.

Grosjean, F. (1985) The Bilingual as a competent but specific speaker-hearer. *Journal of Multilingual and Multicultural Development*, 6, 467–477.

Grosjean, F. (1989) Neurolinguists, beware! The bilingual is not two monolinguals in one person. *Brain and Language*, 36, 3–15.

Gudykunst, W.B. and Kim, Y.Y. (1992) *Communicating with Strangers*, McGraw-Hill, New York.

Gumperz, J.J. (1970) Verbal strategies in multilingual communication, in *Bilingualism and Language Contact*, (ed. J. Alatis), Georgetown University Press, Washington, DC, pp. 129–147.

Gumperz, J.J. (ed.) (1982a) *Language and Social Identity*, Cambridge University Press, Cambridge.

Gumperz, J.J. (1982b) *Discourse Strategies*, Cambridge University Press, Cambridge.

Gumperz, J.J. and Hymes, D. (eds) (1972) *Directions in Sociolinguistics: The Ethnography of Communication*, Holt, Rinehart & Winston, New York.

Habermas, J. (1970) *Towards a Rational Society*, Heinemann, London.

Habermas, J. (1979) *Communication and the Evolution of Society*, (trans. T. McCarthy), Beacon Press, Boston, MA.

Hall, C. (1995) Health advice fails to reach ethnic groups. *The Independent on Sunday*, January 22.

Halliday, M.A.K. (1976) *System and Function in Language*, (ed. G. Kress), Oxford University Press, Oxford.

Harding, S. and Hintikka, M. (eds) (1983) *Discovering Reality: Feminist Perspectives on Epistemology, Methodology and Philosophy of Science*, Dordrecht Reidel, Boston, MA.

Harré, R. (1979) *Social Being: A Theory for Social Psychology,* Blackwell, Oxford.

Harré, R. (1983) *Personal Being: A Theory for Individual Psychology*, Blackwell, Oxford.

Hartley, P. (1993) *Interpersonal Communication*, Routledge, London.

Hawks, J. (1991) Power: A concept analysis. *Journal of Advanced Nursing,* 16, 754–762.

Health Education Authority (1995) *Black and Minority Ethnic Groups in England*, HEA, London.

Hebdige, D. (1975) Reggae, Rastas and Rudies, in *Resistance Through Rituals: Youth Subcultures in Post-War Britain*, (eds S. Hall and T. Jefferson), Hutchinson, London, pp. 135–154.

Henslin, J.M. and Briggs, M.A. (1971) Dramaturgical desexualisation: The sociology of the vaginal examination, in *Studies in the Sociology of Sex*, (eds J.M. Henslin), Appleton-Century-Crofts, New York.

Heritage, J. (1984) *Garfinkel and Ethnomethodology*, Polity Press, Cambridge.

Hewison, A. (1994) The politics of nursing: A framework for analysis. *Journal of Advanced Nursing*, 20, 1170–1175.

Hiro, D. (1973) *Black British, White British*, Pelican, Harmondsworth.

Hockett, C. (1958) *A Course in Modern Linguistics*, Macmillan, New York.

Hodge, R. and Kress, G. (1993) *Language as Ideology*, Routledge, London.

Holmes, J. (1984) Modifying illocutionary force. *Journal of Pragmatics*, 8, 345–365.

Hudson, A. (1989) Changing perspectives: Feminism, gender and social work, in *Radical Social Work Today*, (eds M. Langan and P. Lee), Unwin Hyman, London, pp. 70–96.

Hughes, A. and Trudgill, P. (1978) *English Accents and Dialects: An Introduction to Social and Regional Varieties of British English,* Edward Arnold, London.

Hugman, R. (1991) *Power in Caring Professions*, Macmillan, London.

Hunsaker, P.L. and Alessandra, A.J. (1980) *The Art of Managing People*, Prentice Hall, Englewood Cliffs, NJ.

Husband, C. (1977) A case study in identity maintenance. *European Monographs in Social Psychology*, 13, 310–331.

Husserl, E. (1970) *The Crisis of European Sciences and Transcendental Phenomenology*, North-Western University Press, Evanston, IL.

Hymes, D. (1972) On communicative competence, in *Sociolinguistics*, (eds J.B. Pride and J. Holmes), Penguin, Harmondsworth, pp. 269–293.

Hymes, D. (1977) *Foundations of Sociolinguistics: An Ethnographic Approach,* Tavistock, London.

ILEA (1987) *Language Census,* Inner London Education Authority Research and Statistics, London.

Illich, I. (1973) *Deschooling Society,* Penguin, Harmondsworth.

Illich, I. (1975) *Medical Nemesis,* Calder & Boyars, London.

Ivey, A.E. (1981) Counselling and psychotherapy: Toward a new perspective, in *Cross Cultural Counselling and Psychotherapy,* (eds A.J. Marsella and P.B. Pederson), Pergamon Press, New York.

Ivey, A.E. (1986) *Developmental Therapy,* Jossey-Bass, San Francisco, CA.

Jackson, B. (1975) Black identity development, *Journal of Educational Diversity,* 2, 19–25.

James, W. (1890) *Principles of Psychology,* Holt, New York.

Jenks, C. (1993) *Culture,* Routledge, London.

Jordan, D.W. (1974) *The White Man's Burden,* Oxford University Press, Oxford.

Joyce, J. (1964) *A Portrait of the Artist as a Young Man,* Viking, New York.

Karttunen, F. (1977) Finnish in America: A case study in monogenerational language change, in *Socio-cultural Dimensions of Language Change,* (eds B.G. Blount and M. Sanchez), Academic Press, New York, pp. 173–185.

Katz, J.J. (1981) *Language and Other Abstract Objects,* Rowman & Littlefield, Totowa, NJ.

Kedward, H.R. (1969) *Fascism in Western Europe 1900–45,* Blackie, London.

Keillor, G. (1985) *Lake Wobegone Days,* Faber and Faber, London.

Kelly, G.A. (1955) *The Psychology of Personal Constructs,* Norton, New York.

Kempe, R.S. and Kempe, C.H. (1978) Child Abuse, Open Books, London.

Kleinman, A., Eisenerg, L. and Good, B. (1978) Culture illness and care. *Annals of Internal Medicine,* 88, 252–258.

Kramarae, C. (1982) Gender: How She Speaks, in *Attitudes Toward Language Variation: Social and Applied Contexts,* (eds E.B. Ryan and H. Giles), Edward Arnold, London, pp. 84–89.

Kuhn, T.S. (1970) *The Structure of Scientific Revolutions,* Tavistock, London.

Ladd, P. (1991) The British Sign Language community, in *Multilingualism in the British Isles,* vol. 1, (eds S. Alladina and V. Edwards), Longman, Harlow, pp. 35 48.

Laing, R.D. (1969) *The Divided Self,* Penguin, Harmondsworth.

Laing, R.D. and Esterson, A. (1970) *Sanity, Madness and the Family,* Penguin, Harmondsworth.

Lakoff, R. (1975) *Language and Women's Place,* Harper & Row, New York.

Langan, M. (1993) The rise and fall of social work, in *A Crisis in Care; Challenges to Social Work,* (ed. J. Clarke), Sage Publications, London, pp. 47–68.

Leddy, S. and Pepper, J.M. (1993) *Conceptual Bases of Professional Nursing,* Lippincott, Philadelphia.

Lees, S. (1986) *Losing Out,* Hutchinson, London.

Leininger, M.M. (1967) The culture concept and its relevance to nursing. *Journal of Nursing Education,* 6, 27–37.

Leininger, M.M. (1978) *Transcultural Nursing: Concepts, Theories and Practices,* John Wiley, New York.

Lemert, E.M. (1972) *Human Deviance, Social Problems and Social Control,* Prentice Hall, Englewood Cliffs, NJ.

Linguistic Minorities Project (1985) *The Other Languages of England,* Routledge & Kegan Paul, London.

Lishman, J. (1994) *Communication in Social Work,* Macmillan, Basingstoke.

Littlewood, R. and Lipsedge, M. (1982) *The Aliens and The Alienists: Ethnic Minorities and Psychiatry,* Penguin, Harmondsworth.

Lukes, S. (1974) *Power: A Radical View,* Macmillan, London.

Lukes, S. (1986) *Power,* Blackwell, Oxford.

Luria, A.C. (1973) *The Working Brain,* Penguin, Harmondsworth.

McCrone, J. (1993) *The Myth of Irrationality,* Macmillan, London.

McEwen, W.J. and Greenburg, B.S. (1970) Effects of message intensity on receiver evaluations of source, message and topic. *Journal of Communication,* 20, 340–350.

Mackey, W.F. (1979) Prolegomena to language policy analysis. *Word,* 30, 5.

McLellan, D. (1975) *Marx.* Fontana/Collins, Glasgow.

McLellan, D. (1995) *Ideology.* Open University Press, Buckingham.

Mama, A. (1992) Black women and the British state, in *Racism and Antiracism Inequalities, Opportunities and Policies*, (eds P. Braham, A. Rattansi and P. Skellington), Sage Publications, London, pp. 79–101.

Mann, M. (1983) *Encyclopedia of Sociology,* Macmillan, London.

Mannheim, K. (1959) *Ideology and Utopia,* Harvester, New York.

Manning, N. (ed.) (1985) *Social Problems and Welfare Ideology,* Gower, Aldershot.

Marcos, L.R. and Trujillo, M. (1981) Culture, language and communicative behavior: The psychiatric examination of Spanish Americans, in *Latino Language and Communicative Behavior*, (ed. R.P. Duran), Ablex, Norwood, NJ.

Marcus, L. (1986) Communication concepts and principles, in *Social Work Treatment: Interlocking Theoretical Approaches*, (ed. F.J. Turner), Free Press, New York, pp. 372–399.

Mares, P., Henley, A. and Baxter, C. (1985) *Health Care in Multiracial Britain,* Health Education Council, London.

Marx, K. (1969) The Eighteenth Brumaire of Louis Bonaparte, in *Basic Writings on Politics and Philosophy*, (ed. L.S. Feur), Doubleday, New York, p. 360.

Marx, K. (1975) *Selected Writings*, (ed. D. McLellan), Oxford University Press, Oxford.

Mason, D. (1995) *Race and Ethnicity in Modern Britain*, Oxford University Press, Oxford.

Maxime, J. (1986) Some psychological models of black self-concept, in *Social Work with Black Children and their Families*, (eds S. Ahmed, J. Cheetham and J. Small), Batsford, London, pp. 100–116.

Mayer, J.E. and Timms, N. (1970) *The Client Speaks,* Routledge & Kegan Paul, London.

Mehrley, R.S. and McCroskey, J.C. (1970) Opinionated statements and attitude intensity as predictors of change and source credibility. *Speech Monographs,* 37, 47–52.

Melosh, B. (1982) *The Physician's Hand: Work Culture and Conflict in American Nursing*, Temple University Press, Philadelphia, PA.

Mental Health Act, The. (1983) HMSO, London.

Miles, R. (1989) *Racism,* Routledge & Kegan Paul, London.

Miles, R. (1993) *Racism after 'Race Relations'*, Routledge & Kegan Paul, London.

Miller, N. and Basehart, J. (1969) Source trustworthiness, opinionated statements and responses to persuasive communication. *Speech Monographs,* 36, 1–7.

Miller, N., Maruyama, G., Beaber, R.J. and Valone, K. (1976) Speed of speech and persuasion. *Journal of Personality and Social Psychology,* 34, 615–624.

Min, A. (1993) *Red Azalea,* Victor Gollancz, London.

Mishra, R. (1977) *Society and Social Policy; Theoretical Perspectives on Welfare*, Macmillan, London.

Mosse, G.L. (1966) *The Crisis of German Ideology*, Weidenfield & Nicholson, London.

Mulac, A. (1976) Assessment and application of the Revised Speech Dialect Attitudinal Scale. *Communication Monographs*, 43, 238–245.

Mulac, A. and Lundell, T.L. (1982) An empirical test of the gender-linked language effect in a public speaking setting. *Language and Speech*, 25, 243–256.

Mulac, A. and Lundell, T.L. (1986) Linguistic contributors to the gender-linked language effect in a public speaking setting. *Journal of Language and Social Psychology*, 5, 81–101.

Mulac, A., Lundell, T.L. and Bradac, J.J. (1986) Male/female language differences and attributional consequences in a public speaking situation: Toward an explanation of the gender-linked language effect. *Communication Monographs*, 53, 115–129.

Nahir, M. (1977) The five aspects of language planning: A classification. *Language Problems and Language Planning*, 1, 107–123.

Narayan, U. (1989) Working together across differences, in *Social Work Processes*, (eds B.R. Compton and B. Galaway), Brooks Cole, Pacific Grove, CA, pp. 317–328.

National Health Service and Community Care Act 1990, HMSO, London.

Nelson, J.C. (1980) *Communication Theory and Social Work Practice*, University of Chicago Press, Chicago, IL.

Newbolt, H. (1921) *The Teaching of English in England*, HMSO, London.

Ng, S.H. and Bradac, J.J. (1993) *Power in Language*, Sage Publications, London.

Norman, A. (1985) *Triple Jeopardy: Growing Old in a Second Homeland*, Centre for Policy on Ageing, London.

O'Barr, W. and Atkins, B. (1980) Women's language or powerless language, in *Women and Language in Literature and Society*, (eds S. McConell-Ginet, R. Borker and N. Fulman), Praeger, New York, pp. 93–110.

Ohri, A. (1982) *Community Work and Racism*, Routledge & Kegan Paul, London.

Oliver, M. (1990) *The Politics of Disablement*, Macmillan, London.

Oliver, M. (1994) The politics of disability. *Critical Social Policy*, 11, 21–32.

Omery, A. (1983) Phenomenology: A method for nursing research. *Advanced Nursing Science*, 5, 49–64.

Orem, D. (1985) *Concepts of Nursing*, McGraw Hill, New York.

Owen, M.J. and Holmes, C.A. (1993) Holism in the discourse of nursing. *Journal of Advanced Nursing*, 18, 1688–1695.

Owusu-Bempah, J. (1994) Race, self-identity and social work. *British Journal of Social Work*, 24, 123–136.

Parsons, T. (1937) *The Structure of Social Action*, McGraw-Hill, New York.

Parsons, T. (1960) *Structure and Process in Modern Societies*, Free Press, Chicago, IL.

Pattanayak, D.P. (1991) Foreword, in *Multilingualism in the British Isles*, vol. 1, (eds S. Alladina and V. Edwards), Longman, Harlow, pp. vii–x.

Payne, M. (1991) *Modern Social Work Theory: A Critical Introduction*, Macmillan, Basingstoke.

Pearson, G. (1983) *Hooligan: A History of Respectable Fears*, Macmillan, London.

Pedersen, A. and Pedersen, P. (1989) A cultural grid: A framework for multicultural counselling. *International Journal for the Advancement of Counselling*, 12, 299–307.

Pederson, P.B. (ed.) (1985) *Handbook of Cross-cultural Counseling and Therapy*, Greenwood Press, Westport, CT.

Phillips, D.C. (1977) *Holistic Thought in Social Science,* Stanford University Press, San Francisco, California.

Phillips, P. (1993) A deconstruction of caring. *Journal of Advanced Nursing*, 18, 1554–1558.

Piaget, J.S. (1959) *The Language and Thought of the Child,* Routledge & Kegan Paul, London.

Pilowsky, L. (1994) The pharmacological management of aggressive patients, in *Violence and Health Care Professionals*, (ed. T. Wykes), Chapman & Hall, London, pp. 175–188.

Pincus, A. and Minahan, A. (1973) *Social Work Practice: Model and Method*, Peacock, Itasca, IL.

Ponterotto, J.G. and Casas, J.M. (1987) In search of multi-cultural competence within counselor education programs. *Journal of Counselling and Development*, 65, 430–434.

Porter, S. (1994) New nursing: The road to freedom? *Journal of Advanced Nursing,* 20, 269–274.

Poulantzas, N. (1978) *Political Power and Social Classes,* Verso, London.

Pray, K.L.M. (1949) *Social Work in a Revolutionary Age,* University of Pennsylvania Press, Philadelphia, PA.

Prys, D., Williams, H. and Prys Jones, S. (1993) *Geirfa Gwaith Plant*, University of Wales Press, Cardiff.

Pugh, R. (1992) Lost in translation. *Social Work Today*, 13, 16–17.

Pugh, R. (1994a) *Language Change, Identity and Young People*, paper presented at 40th International Conference of the International Federation of Educative Communities, University of Milwaukee, Milwaukee, WI.

Pugh, R. (1994b) Language policy and social work. *Social Work: The Journal of the American Association of Social Workers,* 39, 432–437.

Pugh, R. and Richards, M. (1996) Speaking out: A practical approach to empowerment. *Practice,* 8, 1.

Raatikainen, R. (1994) Power or the lack of it in nursing care. *Journal of Advanced Nursing*, 19, 424–432.

Rack, P. (1982) *Race, Culture and Mental Disorder,* Tavistock, London.

Rampton, A. (1981) *West Indian Children in our Schools: Interim Report of the Committee of Inquiry into the Education of Children from Ethnic Minority Groups*, HMSO, London.

Rex, J. (1986) *Race and Ethnicity,* Open University Press, Milton Keynes.

Richmond, M. (1917) *Social Diagnosis*, Russell Sage Foundation, New York.

Richmond, M. (1922) *What is Social Casework*, Russell Sage Foundation, New York.

Rivero, Y. and Brice, A. (1994) *Native Language Competence and Second Language Acquisition: An Evaluation of Hispanic Adolescents*, paper presented at 40th International Conference of the International Federation of Educative Communities, University of Milwaukee, Milwaukee, WI.

Rodger, J. (1991) Discourse analysis and social relationships in social work. *British Journal of Social Work*, 21, 63–79.

Rogers, C.R. (1951) *Client-Centred Therapy*, Constable, London.

Rogers, C.R. (1967) *On Becoming a Person: A Therapist's View of Psychotherapy*, Constable, London.

Rogers, M.E. (1970) *An Introduction to the Theoretical Basis of Nursing*, F.A. Davis, Philadelphia, PA.

Rogers, M.E. (1988) Nursing: A science of unitary human beings, in *Conceptual Models for Nursing Practice*, (ed. J. Riehl-Sisca), Appleton & Lange, Norwalk, CT, pp. 181–188.

Rojek, C, Peacock, G. and Collins, S. (1988) *Social Work and Received Ideas*, Routledge, London.

Romaine, S. (1994) *Language in Society*, Oxford University Press, Oxford.

Sacks, H. and Shegloff, E. (1973) Opening up closings. *Semiotica*, 7, 289–327.

Said, E.W. (1993) *Culture and Imperialism*, Chatto & Windus, London.

Saleh, M. (1989) The cultural milieu of counselling. *International Journal for the Advancement of Counselling*, 12, 1, 3–11.

Samovar, L.A. and Porter, R.E, (eds) (1985) *Intercultural Communication: A Reader*, Wadsworth, Belmont, CA.

Sapir, E. (1921) *Language,* Harcourt Brace, New York.

Sapir, E. (1929) The status of linguistics as a science. *Language*, 5, 207–214.

Sashidharan, S. (1989) Schizophrenic – or just black? *Community Care*, 885, 14–15.

Satyamurti, C. (1979) Care and control in Local Authority social work, in *Social Work Welfare and the State*, (eds N. Parry, M. Rustln and C. Satyamurti), Edward Arnold, London, pp. 89–103.

Saussure, F. de (1974) *Course in General Linguistics,* Fontana, London.

Schutz, A. (1972) *The Phenomenology of the Social World,* Heisman, London.

Sharp, K. (1994) Sociology and the nursing curriculum: A note of caution. *Journal of Advanced Nursing*, 20, 391–395.

Shotter, J. (1984) *Social Accountability and Selfhood,* Blackwell, Oxford.

Shotter, J. (1993) *Cultural Politics of Everyday Life*, Open University Press, Buckingham.

Siegal, M. (1990) *Knowing Children: Experiments in Conversation and Cognition,* Lawrence Erlbaum Associates, Hillsdale, NJ.

Simpkin, M. (1979) *Trapped Within Welfare,* Macmillan, London.

Skinner, B.F. (1957) *Verbal Behaviour*, Appleton-Century-Crofts, New York.

Smaje, C. (1995) *Health, Race and Ethnicity*, Kings Fund, London.

Smalley, R.E. (1967) *Theory for Social Work Practice,* Columbia University Press, New York.

Sontag, S. (1978) *Illness as Metaphor,* Farrar, Straus & Giroux, New York.

Sontag, S. (1988) *AIDS and its Metaphors,* Farrar, Straus & Giroux, New York.

Specht, H. and Vickery, A. (1978) *Integrating Social Work Methods*, George Allen & Unwin, London.

Spender, D. (1980) *Man Made Language,* Routledge & Kegan Paul, London.

Spens, W. (1938) *Report of the Consultative Committee on Secondary Education with Special Reference to Grammar Schools and Technical High Schools,* HMSO, London.

Stevenson, B. (1974) *Stevenson's Book of Quotations*, Cassell, London.

Stimson, G. and Webb B. (1993) The face-to-face interaction and after the consultation, in *Health, Welfare and Practice: Reflecting on Roles and Relationships*, (eds J. Walmsley, J. Reynolds, P. Shakespeare and R. Woolfe), Sage Publications, London, pp. 59–64.

Storkey, E. (1991) Race, ethnicity and gender, in *Society and Social Science D 103*, Unit 8, Open University Press, Milton Keynes.

Street, R.L. and Brady, R.M. (1982) Speech rate acceptance ranges as a function of evaluative domain, listener speech rate and communication context. *Communication Monographs,* 49, 290–308.

Street, R.L., Brady, R.M. and Putman, W.B. (1983) The influence of speech rate stereotypes and rate similarity on listener's evaluations of speakers. *Journal of Language and Social Psychology*, 2, 37–56.

Sue, D.W. and Sue, D. (1990) *Counselling the Culturally Different: Theory and Practice,* Wiley-Interscience, New York.

Swain, J., Finkelstein, V., French, S. and Oliver, M. (1993) *Disabling Barriers – Enabling Environments*, Sage Publications, London.

Swann, Lord (1985) *Education for All: The Report of the Committee of Inquiry into the Education of Children from Ethnic Minority Groups*, HMSO, London.

Szasz, T.S. (1972) *The Myth of Mental Illness,* Paladin, London.

Tajfel, H. (1974) Social identity and intergroup behaviour. *Social Science Information*, 13, 65–93.

Tajfel, H. (1978) *Differentiation Between Social Groups: Studies in the Social Psychology of Intergroup Relations,* Academic Press, London.

Tannen, D. (1986) *That's Not What I Meant!: How Conversational Style Makes or Breaks Your Relations With Others*, Ballantine, New York.

Taylor, G. (1993) Challenges from the margins, in *A Crisis in Care: Challenges to Social Work*, (ed. J. Clarke), Sage Publications, London, pp. 103–146.

Taylor, I., Walton, P. and Young, J. (1973) *The New Criminology: For a Social Theory of Deviance,* Routledge & Kegan Paul, London.

Taylor, W. (1981) *Probation and After-Care in a Multi-Racial Society*, Commission on Racial Equality, London.

Thomas, V. and Dines, A. (1994) The health care needs of ethnic minority groups: Are nurses and individuals playing their part? *Journal of Advanced Nursing*, 20, 802–808.

Thompson, N. (1993) *Anti-Discriminatory Practice*, BASW/Macmillan, London.

Thomson, R. and Scott, S. (1991) *Learning About Sex: Young Women and the Social Construction of Sexual Identity,* Tufnel Press, London.

Tizard, B. and Hughes, M. (1984) *Young Children Learning,* Fontana, London.

Trudgill, P. (1983) *Sociolinguistics,* Penguin, Harmondsworth.

Ussher, J. (1991) *Women's Madness: Misogyny or Mental Illness*, Harvester Wheatsheaf, Hemel Hempstead.

Utting, W. (1991) *Children in the Public Care,* HMSO, London.

Van der Veer, R. and Valsiner, J. (1991) *Understanding Vygotsky: A Quest for Synthesis,* Blackwell, Oxford.

Velasquez, J., Vigil, M.E. and Benavides, E. (1989) A framework for establishing social work relationships across racial/ethnic lines, in *Social Work Processes*, (eds B.R. Compton and B. Galaway), Brooks Cole, Pacific Grove, CA, pp. 312–316.

Vinge, L. (1975) *The Five Senses: Studies in a Literary Tradition*, Lund, Sweden.

Volosinov, V.N. (1976) *Freudanism: A Marxist Critique*, Academic Press, New York.

Vygotsky, L.S. (1962) *Thought and Language,* MIT Press, Cambridge, MA.

Walmsley, J., Reynolds, J., Shakespeare, P. and Woolfe, R. (1993) *Health, Welfare and Practice: Reflecting on Roles and Relationships*, Sage Publications, London.

Ward, D. and Mullender, A. (1993) Empowerment and oppression: An indissoluble pairing for contemporary social work, in *Health, Welfare and Practice: Reflecting on Roles and Relationships*, (eds J. Walmsley, J. Reynolds, P. Shakespeare and R. Woolfe), Sage Publications, London, pp. 147–154.

Watson, J.B. (1924) *Psychology from the Standpoint of a Behaviourist,* J.B. Lippincott, Philadelphia, PA.

Webb, B. (1993) Trauma and tedium: An account of living on a children's ward, in *Health, Welfare and Practice: Reflecting on Roles and Relationships*, (eds J. Walmsley, J. Reynolds, P. Shakespeare and R. Woolfe), Sage Publications, London, pp. 184–189.

Webb, D. (1981) Themes and continuities in radical and traditional social work. *British Journal of Social Work*, 11, 143–158.

Wells, G. (1987) *The Meaning Makers: Children Using Language and Using Language to Learn*, Hodder & Stoughton, London.

Welsh Language Act (1967) HMSO, Cardiff.

Welsh Language Act (1993) HMSO, Cardiff.

Welsh Office (1992) *Welsh Social Survey,* HMSO, Cardiff.

Westley, B.H. and MacLean, M.S. (1957) A conceptual model for communication research. *Journalism Quarterly*, 34, 31–38.

White, R. (1985) *Political Issues in Nursing*, vol. 1, John Wiley, Chichester.

White, R. (1986) *Political Issues in Nursing*, vol. 2, John Wiley, Chichester.

White, R. (1988) *Political Issues in Nursing*, vol. 3, John Wiley, Chichester.

Whorf, B.L. (1976) *Language, Thought and Reality: Selected Writings of Benjamin Lee Whorf* (ed. J. Carroll), MIT Press, Cambridge, MA.

Widdicombe, S. and Wooffitt, R. (1995) *The Language of Youth Subcultures*, Harvester Wheatsheaf, Hemel Hempstead.

Wilding, P. (1982) *Professional Power and Social Welfare,* Routledge & Kegan Paul, London.

Wilkins, H. (1993) Transcultural nursing: A selective review of the literature, 1985–1991. *Journal of Advanced Nursing*, 18, 602–612.

Williams, D.M. (1989) Political theory and individualistic health promotion. *Advances in Nursing Science*, 12, 14–25.

Williams, G. (1992) *Sociolinguistics: A Sociological Critique*, Routledge, London.

Williams, G.A. (1985) *When Was Wales?*, Penguin, London.

Williams, G.A. (1988a) Beginnings of Radicalism, in *The Remaking of Wales in the 18th Century*, (eds T. Herbert and G.E. Jones), University of Wales Press, Cardiff, pp. 111–147.

Williams, H. (1988b) *A Social Work Vocabulary,* University of Wales Press, Cardiff.

Williams, H. (1994) Gwaith Cymdeithasol a'r Iaith Gymraeg/Social Work and the Welsh Language, in *Gwaith Cymdeithasol a'r Iaith Gymraeg/Social Work and the Welsh Language/Social Work and the Welsh Language,* CCETSW, Cardiff.

Williams, R.H., Williams, H. and Davis, E. (eds) (1994) *Gwaith Cymdeithasol a'r Iaith Gymraeg/Social Work and the Welsh Language*, CCETSW, Cardiff.

Wolf, S. (1994) *The Treatment of Sexually Aggressive Children and Young People*, paper presented at the NEWI Child Protection Conference, Wrexham, Wales.

Wrong, D. (1961) The oversocialized conception of man in modern sociology. *American Sociological Review*, 26, 183–193.

Zborowski, M. (1958) Cultural components in responses to pain, in *Patients, Physicians, and Illness*, (ed. E.G. Jago), Free Press, Glencoe, IL, pp. 256–268.

Zentella, A.C. (1987) Language and female identity, in *Women and Language in Transition*, (ed. J. Penfield), SUNY Press, New York.

Zulueta, F. de (1990) Bilingualism and family therapy. *Journal of Family Therapy*, 12, 225–265.

Index